Methotrexate in the Treatment of Autoimmune Diseases –

Modern Concepts in Rheumatology, Dermatology and Gastroenterology

UNI-MED

UNI-MED Verlag AG
Bremen - London - Boston

Müller-Ladner, Ulf:
Methotrexate in the Treatment of Autoimmune Diseases – Modern Concepts in Rheumatology, Dermatology and Gastroenterology/Ulf Müller-Ladner.-
1st edition - Bremen: UNI-MED, 2025
ISBN 978-3-8374-1676-3

Printed in Europe

MEDICINE - STATE OF THE ART

UNI-MED Verlag AG, one of the leading medical publishing companies in Germany, presents its highly successful series of scientific textbooks, covering all medical subjects. The authors are specialists in their fields and present the topics precisely, comprehensively, and with the facility of quick reference in mind. The books will be most useful for all doctors who wish to keep up to date with the latest developments in medicine.

The publisher would like to thank the company medac for supporting the production of this edition. The publisher assures that the industry partner could not influence the content of the book in any way, especially not therapy recommendations.

Preface

Methotrexate is still the anchor drug for the majority of inflammatory rheumatic diseases, and the body of data supporting its use is still growing. To illustrate the current and future value of methotrexate in the treatment algorithms and therapeutic approaches, experts in the field have compiled the state-of-the-art knowledge for immediate use in practice and clinic.

Giessen/Bad Nauheim, December 2024 *Ulf Müller-Ladner*

Authors

Editors

Prof. Dr. Ulf Müller-Ladner
Justus-Liebig-Universität Giessen
Abt. Rheumatologie und Klinische Immunologie
Kerckhoff-Klinik GmbH
Benekestraße 2-8
61231 Bad Nauheim

Co-Authors

Prof. Dr. Martin Aringer
Universitätsklinikum Carl Gustav Carus Dresden
an der Technischen Universität Dresden
Medizinische Klinik und Poliklinik III
Leiter des Bereiches Rheumatologie
Fetscherstraße 74
01307 Dresden

Chapter 6.

Prof. Dr. Christoph Baerwald
Universitätsklinikum Leipzig AöR
Department für Innere Medizin, Neurologie und Dermatologie
Klinik für Gastroenterologie und Rheumatologie
Leiter der Sektion Rheumatologie
Liebigstraße 20
04103 Leipzig

Chapter 3.

Prof. Dr. Christoph Fiehn
Medical Center Baden-Baden
Innere Medizin/Rheumatologie
Beethovenstraße 2
76530 Baden-Baden

Chapter 2.

Prof. Dr. Rebecca Fischer-Betz
Universitätsklinikum Düsseldorf
Moorenstraße 5
40225 Düsseldorf

Chapter 11.

Dr. Walter Hermann
Justus-Liebig-Universität Giessen
Abt. Rheumatologie und Klinische Immunologie
Kerckhoff-Klinik GmbH
Benekestraße 2-8
61231 Bad Nauheim

Chapter 1.

Prof. Dr. Nicolas Hunzelmann
Klinik für Dermatologie
Uniklinik Köln
Kerpener Straße 62
50937 Cologne

Chapter 8.

Prof. Dr. Gernot Keyßer
Universitätsklinikum Halle (Saale)
Universitätsklinik und Poliklinik für Innere Medizin II
Leiter des Arbeitsbereiches Rheumatologie
Ernst-Grube-Straße 40
06120 Halle (Saale)

Chapter 10.

Prof. Dr. Klaus Krüger
Praxiszentrum St. Bonifatius
St. Bonifatius Straße 5
81541 Munich

Chapter 4.

Prof. Dr. Torsten Kucharzik
Klinik für Allgemeine Innere Medizin und Gastroenterologie
Klinikum Lüneburg
Bögelstraße. 1
21339 Lüneburg

Chapter 9.

Prof. Dr. Kirsten Minden
Deutsches Rheumaforschungszentrum Berlin und Universitätsmedizin Charité Berlin, Klinik für Rheumatologie und Immunologie
Charitéplatz 1
10117 Berlin

Chapter 7.

Dr. Daniela Neumayer
Klinik für Dermatologie
Uniklinik Köln
Kerpener Straße 62
50937 Cologne

Chapter 8.

Dr. Siegfried Wassenberg
Rheumazentrum Ratingen
and
Rheumaklinik - Fachklinik 360°
Rosenstraße 2
40882 Ratingen

Chapter 5.

Dr. Inga Wellstein
Universitätsklinikum Leipzig AöR
Department für Innere Medizin, Neurologie und Dermatologie
Klinik für Gastroenterologie und Rheumatologie
Leiter der Sektion Rheumatologie
Liebigstraße 20
04103 Leipzig

Chapter 3.

Contents

1. Introduction

1.1. The current role of methotrexate in the treatment of rheumatoid arthritis

Following its wider introduction as a new standard therapy for rheumatoid arthritis (RA) in the mid-1980s, methotrexate (MTX) has proven to be equivalent or superior to other standard therapies in comparative trials. It inhibits radiological progression, induces healing of erosions and has a life-prolonging effect. In long-term studies, MTX showed a lower discontinuation rate and thus a longer "drug survival rate" than other disease-modifying substances.

> To date, MTX is the most important and most frequently prescribed standard therapy for RA worldwide and is recommended by most professional medical societies as the primary DMARD (disease-modifying antirheumatic drug). It owes this status to
>
> - its good efficacy and relatively low toxicity,
> - its simple method of administration, either oral or parenteral, and
> - the ability to adjust the dose to a wide range of individual needs.

MTX has also been established as a central component of various combination treatment regimens for RA as it enhances the effectivity of other DMARDs. It is indispensable in combination with TNF inhibitors. TNF inhibition proves to be more clinically effective in combination with MTX than a monotherapy with MTX or biologics. MTX also inhibits the formation of antibodies that reduce the half-life and the effective dose level of a biologic. Registry data also show increased adherence to therapy among patients treated with biologics (62).

In addition, MTX is also the cornerstone of treatment for psoriatic arthritis (PsA) and juvenile idiopathic arthritis (JIA). Finally, it has been and still is used for inflammatory myopathies, connective tissue diseases, such as SLE and various vasculitides, as a substitute for other immunomodulators and/or because of its steroid-sparing effect.

1.2. History of methotrexate treatment

1.2.1. The beginnings

In the 1940s, the importance of folic acid for the function of hematopoietic cells was recognized. It was deduced that the inhibition of folic acid should therefore be suitable in tumor therapy. The folic acid analogue aminopterin, synthesized in 1947, had a cytostatic effect through competitive inhibition of folic acid (1) and was successfully used in childhood leukemia as early as 1948 (2). In the same year, the less toxic folic acid antagonist 4-amino-10-methyl-folic acid, methotrexate, was synthesized (3).

In 1951, Jimenez-Diaz et al. published the use of the cytostatic agent nitrogen mustard in RA (4). In the same year, Gubner (5) reported on the aminopterin treatment of eight patients with chronic joint inflammation. With daily oral administration of 1-2 mg of aminopterin, the symptoms of five RA patients improved rapidly, and in one patient with PsA, the psoriasis eruptions healed rapidly. While the investigations into rheumatic diseases were initially not pursued further due to the dawning era of steroids, Rees adopted aminopterin in daily doses of 0.5-1 mg for the treatment of severe cases of psoriasis and reported significant improvement in around 80% of 171 and 229 patients, respectively, in 1954 and 1959 (6, 7). In the following years, MTX at daily doses of 2.5 mg proved to be just as effective but less toxic than aminopterin in the treatment of psoriasis (8, 9).

Since single high doses were less toxic in animal experiments than repeated low doses (10) and the toxicity appeared to be directly proportional to the duration of exposure (11), Roenigk recommended a single weekly oral dose of 25 mg in 1965 (12), if necessary administered in three equal doses with 12-hour intervals (13).

Since the early 1960s, MTX has been prescribed on a large scale in the USA for psoriasis, and was approved for this indication by the FDA in 1972. Its effectivity in PA was confirmed with a double-blind study in 1964 (14).

After successfully treating experimental thyroiditis in guinea pigs (15), Miescher and Riethmüller also used MTX in connective tissue diseases, particularly SLE, for the first time (16).

1.2.2. Early studies for rheumatoid arthritis

In 1967, Gross et al. (17) from Zurich reported on significant clinical and blood chemical improvements in patients with highly active "treatment-refractory" RA treated with 50(!) mg MTX per week intravenously. Due to some severe side effects, the Zurich Rheumatology Clinic tabooed MTX.

In 1972, Hoffmeister reported on 29 patients with highly active RA whose joint symptoms improved significantly with 10-15 mg MTX orally per week, but mostly worsened again when the dose was reduced to less than 10 mg/week (18). By 1982, he had observed a "marked improvement" in 58% of 78 patients, including a "complete remission" in 36% (19).

These and other publications of retrospective studies, open prospective and finally placebo-controlled studies aroused a new interest among rheumatologists in MTX treatment in the early 1980s and stimulated its research and application.

In 1980, two pilot studies were published from Cleveland and Seattle, where experience with MTX treatment of RA had apparently been gained for some time - unnoticed by the public.

In six previously treatment-resistant RA patients, Wilke observed a significant reduction in disease activity after 6 and 12 weeks of treatment with 7.5 mg MTX per week orally (20). In 1980, Willkens described a significant reduction in the number of affected joints and ESR in 32 patients taking 7.5-15 mg MTX per week (21), and in 1982 long-term results over 15 years in 150 RA patients with a success rate of 85% with weekly doses between 5 and 20 mg MTX (22).

Unaware of the experience with MTX in the US, we have been using MTX for RA in Ratingen since 1979 following a positive report on the treatment of a patient with PsA. After several inquiries to the manufacturer Lederle, including the US headquarters, we were strongly advised not to use MTX for rheumatic diseases: it was a tumor therapeutic and there was no experience with rheumatic diseases. In general, we started the therapy without folic acid supplementation intravenously with weekly doses of 25 or 15 mg, depending on body weight, age, general condition, concomitant diseases, kidney function, etc. We did not see a high rate of side effects. After 1-3 months, we then switched to oral medication at the same dose and increased the dose accordingly if it was less effective. At first we viewed MTX primarily as a highly potent anti-inflammatory agent and used it in addition to a standard therapeutic agent, especially gold, to stop flares in highly active cases. As early as 1982, Karger et al. described a significant reduction in disease activity, steroid requirements and ESR in 20 of 28 patients with highly active RA who were prospectively treated with 10-25 mg MTX weekly after 1 to 3 years. Seven patients went into remission (23).

It must be emphasized that in the experimental phase of MTX treatment, the majority of cases treated were not only active but also "treatment-refractory" and at an advanced stage, which made it all the more difficult to achieve dramatic success. In a long-term study, 69% of the 31 patients were in anatomical stages III and IV according to Steinbrocker. After 3 years, their clinical and laboratory data had improved significantly and steroid consumption was significantly reduced (24).

Weinstein et al. observed 15 of the original 21 patients with RA for 42 months with MTX doses of between 7.5 and 15 mg per week. The improvement in clinical data and ESR was highly significant. Three patients went into remission (25).

> Pilot studies and small prospective open studies in the early 1980s found impressive improvements in disease activity with a simultaneous reduction in the prednisone dose during MTX treatment.

1.2.3. Placebo-controlled short-term studies

In order to confirm the clinical observations, several randomized, double-blind, placebo-controlled studies were carried out in the mid-1980s. These, too, were all chronic advanced "treatment-refractory" cases.

In the treatment of 189 patients with oral doses of 7.5 to 15 mg per week over 18 weeks, MTX proved to be significantly superior to placebo in all parameters examined. The number of tender joints fell by 34%, the number of swollen joints by 27%, the ESR by 29%, grip strength increased by 33%, and morning stiffness improved by 40% (26, 27). A 24-week crossover study in 35 patients with 7.5-15 mg per week showed a 50% improvement in the pain and joint swelling index in 54% and 39% of the patients, respectively. The improvement usually began after just three weeks of treatment. After switching from MTX to placebo, an arthritis flare was regularly observed (28). On the basis of these two studies, the FDA approved MTX for the treatment of RA in 1988. The results of two other placebo-controlled studies with intramuscular application of MTX were similarly convincing (29, 30) (☞ Table 1.1).

Improvements (%) using MTX

A meta-analysis of the 4 studies showed a reduction in the number of tender and swollen joints by 39% and 26%, respectively, for MTX compared to placebo (31).

Furst (32) found a significant ($p<0.05$) linear improvement in efficacy comparing placebo, 5 mg/m² MTX and 10 mg/m² MTX per week in 46 patients who were treated double-blind on an outpatient basis for 16 weeks. Interestingly, after two weeks of inpatient pre-treatment, there was a highly significant improvement in 9 of the 11 efficacy parameters in the placebo group as well as in the two verum groups.

Russell observed a significant improvement after just 3-6 weeks of weekly intramuscular doses of 10 mg (n=17) or 25 mg (n=14) compared to a placebo group (n=17) without any noticeable differences in effectivity between the two MTX doses (33). A dose-effect relationship is now generally accepted.

Intravenous weekly doses of 15-25 mg (34) and 50 mg (35) proved to act very fast and be highly effective.

> Placebo-controlled studies showed a significant superiority of MTX in all parameters and thus confirmed the results of the open studies.

1.2.4. Comparative studies with rarely used standard therapeutic agents

Comparison with Auranofin®

Two large US multicenter studies achieved different results when comparing auranofin® (AF) (oral gold preparation) with MTX. In the comparative study by Weinblatt (36), 281 patients were treated for 36 weeks with either 7.5 mg MTX per week, increased to 15 mg in 43%, or 6 mg AF daily, increased to 9 mg in 41%. In both groups, all clinical parameters improved significantly ($p<0.01$), but significantly more and more quickly with MTX. Side effects and treatment discontinuations were less common with MTX.

In the three-arm multicenter study by Williams (37), no statistically significant differences in clinical efficacy were evident between 6 mg AF daily (n=115) and 7.5 mg MTX weekly (n=114) over a treatment period of 48 weeks. However, the ESR improved more in the MTX group. The number of treatment discontinuations due to side effects was the same at 16 and 17 respectively, and discon-

Author	Year	n	Weekly dose	Application	Duration (weeks)	Joint Index Pain	Joint Index Swelling	ESR	Grip strength	Morning stiffness
Williams (26)	1985	189	7.5-15 mg	oral	18	34%	27%	29%	33%	40%
Weinblatt (28)	1985	35	7.5-15 mg *crossover*	oral	24	54%	39%	–	30%	73%
Andersen (29)	1985	15	5.0-25 mg	IM	26	30%	18%	22%	12%	67%
Thompson (30)	1984	48	10.0-25 mg *crossover*	IM	6	52%	64%	46%	15%	70%
Metaanalysis (31)	1987	287	7.5-22 mg	oral/ IM	18	39%	26%	15%	28%	46%

Table 1.1: Placebo-controlled short-term studies in "treatment-resistant" patients using MTX. Significant improvement of all parameters compared to placebo. The percentage of improvement is given.

tinuation due to ineffectiveness was higher in the AF group (n=15) than in the MTX group (n=8).

In a controlled study, 7.5-15 mg MTX per week was more effective and better tolerated than 6-9 mg AF per day. Another study found no significant differences between 7.5 mg MTX per week and 6 mg AF per day. However, MTX improved the ESR more and showed fewer treatment discontinuations due to insufficient effect.

Comparison with parenteral gold

Three smaller comparative studies between parenteral gold (50 mg aurothiomalate (ATM) per week) and MTX (10-15 mg per week) over 6 to 12 months showed significant improvements in all clinical parameters with no significant difference between the groups but lower toxicity with MTX (38-40).

A randomized, double-blind study conducted in two German centers (Ratingen and Bad Abbach) compared 50 mg ATM with 15 mg MTX per week intramuscularly in 174 patients with early erosive RA, i.e. with erosions but without joint destruction (Larsen stage >3) with a mean disease duration of 11 months (41). Even after discontinuation of therapy, all patients were followed up quarterly. The ITT and Completer analyses showed a significant improvement of >50% in all six clinical variables including activities of daily living (ADL), ESR and CRP with no significant difference between the groups (☞ Figure 1.1) (41).

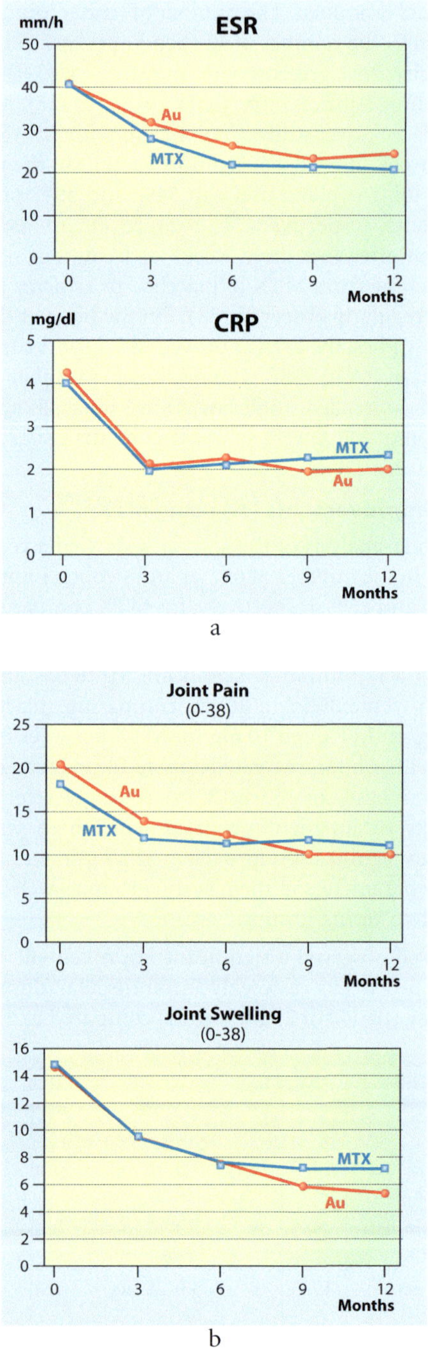

Figure 1.1a+b: Sedimentation rate (ESR) and CRP (**a**) as well as number of painful and swollen joints (**b**) in the first 12 months of the Au/MTX study. Significant improvement in both groups by about 50% with no significant difference between the groups (41).

10 patients (11.5%) in the MTX group and 21 patients (24.1%) in the gold group achieved clinical remission, defined as absence of joint swelling, ESR <20 mm and no steroid administration within the last 3 months. Significant improvement (>50% reduction in the number of swollen joints and ESR) was achieved by 68% of the MTX group and 76% of the gold group (p>0.05). The mean prednisone dose decreased from 4.5 mg to 0.7 mg daily using MTX and from 2.9 to 0.3 mg using gold (☞ Table 1.2) (41).

After the one-year double-blind phase, the study was continued openly for two years while maintaining the MTX dose of 15 mg IM per week, but with the gold dose halved to 50 mg ATM every 2 weeks. The activity parameters continued to improve to the same extent in both groups. Clinical remissions were achieved in 33% (MTX) and 38% (ATM) (ITT analysis). A significant clinical improvement in the activity parameters of >50% was achieved in 78% of the patients treated with MTX and 87% of the patients treated with gold (42). 16% of the MTX patients and 53% of the gold patients discontinued treatment due to side effects (p=0.0001). The time to discontinuation was significantly shorter with gold than with MTX (☞ Figure 1.2) (42).

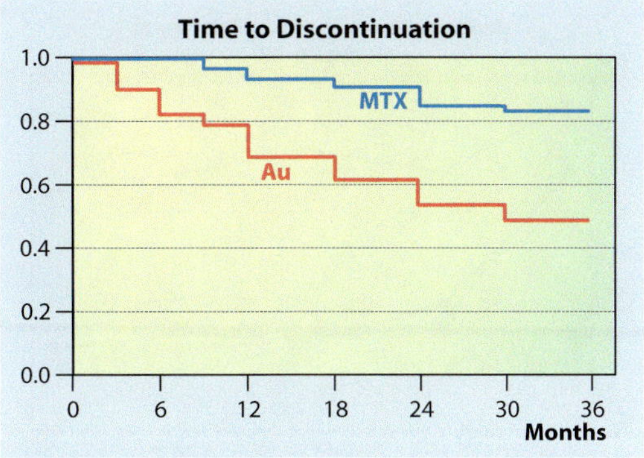

Figure 1.2: Time to discontinuation of therapy due to toxicity in the Au/MTX study. Each grroup of 87 patients was treated with either MTX or aurothiomalate. Kaplan-Meier curve. The time to discontinuation was significantly longer using MTX (p<0.0001) (42).

Of the 128 patients recruited for this study in Ratingen, complete data were documented for 117 (88%) over up to 6 years after the start of therapy (43). In 57% of those who discontinued MTX, the discontinuation was due to side effects, and in 43% due to ineffectivity. After 6 years, the clinical outcome (improvement in all parameters by 40-70%) in those who discontinued gold therapy was comparable to that of those who completed gold and MTX therapy (43). In those affected by gold rash, the arthritis improved particularly quickly and impressively (☞ Figure 1.3) (43).

	MTX (n=73)				ATM (n=53)			
	0	6	12	p	0	6	12	p
Swollen joints (0-38)	14.9 ± 6.5	8.0 ± 6.7	7.6 ± 6.9	*	14.6 ± 7.2	7.5 ± 7.7	6.1 ± 7.5	*
Grip strength right hand (bar)	0.3 ± 0.2	0.5 ± 0.2	0.5 ± 0.3	*	0.3 ± 0.2	0.4 ± 0.3	0.5 ± 0.2	*
FFbH (0-100%)	69.1 ± 19.2	81.1 ± 25.7	78.4 ± 19.3	*	72.3 ± 20.6	79.8 ± 16.6	80.7 ± 20.7	*
ESR (mm/h)	41.5 ± 24.6	22.8 ± 19.8	21.1 ± 16.2	*	41.0 ± 25.7	26.0 ± 27.4	23.4 ± 29.8	*
CRP (mg/dl)	4.1 ± 3.6	2.2 ± 2.6	2.5 ± 3.2	*	4.3 ± 3.9	2.2 ± 3.0	2.1 ± 2.9	

Table 1.2: Course of therapy with MTX and gold over one year (Au/MTX study) – Completer analysis (41).
* = statistically significant p<0.05; FFbH = Hannover Functional Questionnaire (100% = normal function).

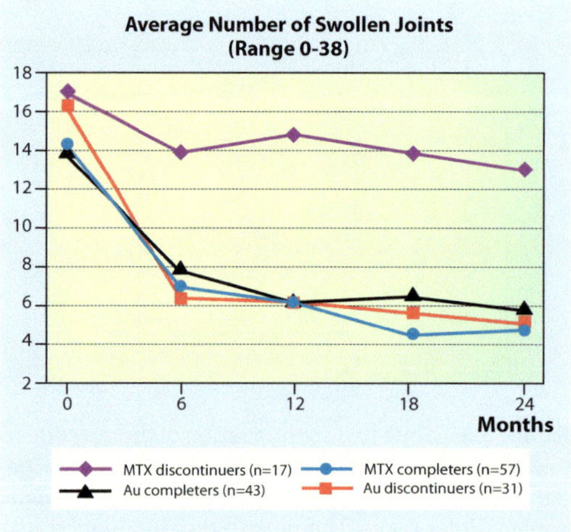

Figure 1.3: Number of swollen joints over 24 months in completers and discontinuers of the Au/MTX study from one center (43).

> Assuming optimal dosage of both substances, MTX is almost equal to parenteral gold in terms of clinical efficacy and induction of remission. Significantly more patients discontinued treatment with gold compared to MTX, almost exclusively because of a gold rash. Patients with rashes also responded particularly well to the therapy in the long term.

Comparison with azathioprine

42 patients with long-term active RA were treated in a double-blind study for 24 weeks with 100 mg azathioprine (AZA) daily or 10 mg MTX weekly. All nine clinical variables improved statistically significantly in both groups, tending to improve more quickly and more significantly with MTX (44).

In a second double-blind study, 33 patients were treated with 100-150 mg AZA and 31 patients with 7.5-15 mg MTX. The discontinuation rate was significantly higher in the AZA group. The improvement in the number of swollen joints, the pain index and the ESR was significantly greater after 24 and 48 weeks using MTX compared to AZA (45).

> Studies showed MTX to be more effective and better tolerated than AZA.

1.2.4.1. Meta-analysis of early DMARD comparative studies

In 1990, Felson published a meta-analysis of studies comparing standard drug treaments with each other or with placebo, in which a total of 3,957 patients were included. He came to the conclusion that MTX was significantly more effective than AF and comparable to D-penicillamine and intramuscular gold (46). However, meta-analyses should be interpreted with caution, as study populations (inclusion and exclusion criteria, duration, activity and severity of the disease) and the different treatment regimens (including dosage, concomitant therapy with corticosteroids) are often difficult to compare.

> A meta-analysis found MTX to be equal to parenteral gold and D-penicillamine, and superior to AF and AZA.

1.2.5. Assessment of potential methotrexate toxicity

Particular attention was paid to potential side effects of MTX. A report by Scandinavian dermatologists on the occurrence of liver cirrhosis during the treatment of psoriasis with MTX (47, 48), albeit with doses spread over the week and higher alcohol consumption, made liver toxicity the most feared complication of MTX treatment. Liver biopsies before and during long-term treatment with MTX (49, 50) showed no deterioration in the histological findings during therapy and only mild fibrosis after long-term treatment (51). Elevations in TA occurred mainly in the initial phase of treatment (52) and were rare during long-term treatment (53). With the extension of the indication to include less seriously ill patients, it became apparent that "clinically important" side effects with regard to other organs were also rare. Good efficacy and tolerability made MTX the drug with the longest treatment adherence in Rheumatology.

The weekly dose of 7.5 mg, which was initially introduced as standard in the USA, was gradually increased to 15-20 mg. The discontinuation rate was further reduced by routine folic acid supplementation leading to a reduction in gastrointestinal side effects. This also made it possible to further increase MTX doses. However, there is evidence that the additional folic acid impairs the effectiveness of MTX (54).

MTX has become the most widely used DMARD worldwide. According to the German National Database (Kerndokumentation, www.dfrz.de) released in 2021, 53% of RA patients are being treated with MTX (53% orally, 47% subcutaneously), and 40% of PsA patients received MTX. In view of the individual variation and incomplete absorption of MTX, there is an increasing switch from oral to subcutaneous administration if the effectivity is insufficient. A comparison of both forms of administration was clearly in favor of subcutaneous administration (55).

> The feared liver toxicity of MTX could be mitigated by long-term monitoring of TA and serial liver biopsies. The tolerability in general has also proved to be satisfactory.

In 1991, MTX was also approved for the treatment of RA by the German Federal Health Office. Despite its high esteem as a DMARD, the finding later obtained in several three-arm studies was very surprising: MTX monotherapy was in no way less effective than monotherapy with one of the highly praised biologics. Interestingly, the combination with MTX was clearly superior to both monotherapies (56-58) and made MTX indispensable as a combination partner with biologics. MTX also proved to be an anchor drug in the treatment of RA in other combination therapies (59).

1.3. Recommendations and guidelines for the treatment of rheumatoid arthritis

The update of the EULAR RA Management Recommendations from 2023 (63) retained the key statements on MTX therapy from 2014: Treatment of RA with DMARDs should be initiated and monitored immediately after diagnosis by a rheumatologist as the responsible specialist. The aim of therapy is remission or a state of low disease activity. MTX should be used as the first-line drug. A dose of 0.3 mg per kg body weight per week should be aimed for within 4-6 weeks. This means that the target dose should usually be around 20-25 mg per week. Additional administration of folic acid is required. If MTX is contraindicated due to kidney or liver disease, leflunomide or sulfasalazine can be prescribed as an alternative. If the disease is still active, follow-up examinations must take place at intervals of 1-3 months and can be reduced to intervals of 6-12 months once the treatment goal has been achieved. If no effectivity is evident after 3 months or the treatment goal has not been achieved after 6 months, treatment must be adjusted. If the result is unsatisfactory, combination with other conventional or biological DMARDs must be considered. GCs can be used at the start of therapy to bridge the time until the DMARDs become effective. They should then be reduced and removed from therapy as quickly as possible (the aim should be to end corticoid therapy after 3 months at the latest). In the German S2e guideline on drug therapy for RA (64), which was drawn up in 2018, MTX monotherapy is recommended as the first standard therapy, unchanged from the S1 guideline from 2012. An advantage of a primary combination of several DMARDs cannot yet be proven. Treatment should ideally be started within 12 weeks of the onset of symptoms, as soon as the diagnosis of RA is made, possibly even before RA is confirmed. An "optimization" of MTX treatment is recommended after just three months if the treatment goal has not been achieved. "Optimized" monotherapy means higher dosage or switching to parenteral administration.

> After 12 weeks of DMARD therapy, a 50% improvement in the composite score (usually DAS28) should be achieved, and after 24 weeks the treatment goal should be achieved (65).

At the start of therapy, GC should be given in addition to MTX. An initial starting dose of 30 mg prednisolone equivalent per day is recommended. A reduction to a low dose should then be aimed for within 8 weeks.

Every bDMARD and tsDMARD should be combined with MTX if possible.

Comment on the German S1 guideline

The need to combine MTX with GC in all cases must be questioned. The new diagnostic ACR/EULAR criteria also include patients who will not develop chronic joint inflammation. In the guideline, this is called "over-diagnosis". In addition, GC overshadows the DMARD effect, making the actual MTX effect difficult to estimate. In DMARD studies, which are usually carried out on highly active patients, a maximum of 7.5 or 10 mg GC per day is therefore permitted.

In the opinion of the editors, the dangers of GC are underestimated: they have a stimulating and euphoric effect and are therefore addictive. Weaning is difficult because adrenal cortex insufficiency develops and GC are needed to replace the reduced production in the body. GC have been identified in many studies as independent predictors of increased mortality. For this reason, the start of any GC administration should be viewed critically and should not be done automatically. In many cases, it will be possible to achieve rapid and sufficient therapeutic success without GC.

1.4. References

1. Seeger DR, Smith JM Jr, Hultquist ME. Antagonist for pteroyl-glutamic acid. J Am Chem Soc 1947; 69: 2567

2. Farber S, Diamond LK, Mercer RD, Sylvester RF, Wolff JA. Temporary remissions in acute leucemia in children produced by folic acid antagonist, 4-aminopteroyl-glutamic acid (aminopterin). N Engl J Med 1948; 238: 787-93

3. Smith JM Jr.,Cosulich DB, Hultquist ME, Seeger DR. The chemistry of certain pteroylglutamic acid antagonists. Trans NY Acad Sci 1948; 10: 82-3

4. Jimenez-Diaz C, Garcia E, Merchante A, Perianes J. Treatment of rheumatoid arthritis with nitrogen mustard. J Amer Med Ass 1951; 147: 1418

5. Gubner R, August S, Ginsberg V. Therapeutic suppression of tissue reactivity. II. Effect of aminopterin in rheumatoid arthritis and psoriasis. Am J Med Sci 1951; 221: 176-82

6. Rees RB, Bennett JH, Bostick WL. Aminopterin for psoriasis. Arch Dermatol 1955; 72: 133-43

7. Rees RB,Bennett JH. Further observations on aminopterin for psoriasis.J Invest Dermatol 1959; 32: 61-6

8. Edmundson WF, Gay WB. Treatment of psoriasis with folic acid antagonists. Arch Dermatol 1958; 78:200-3

9. Rees RB, Bennett JH. Methotrexate versus aminopterin for psoriasis. Arch Dermatol 1961; 83: 970-2

10. Ferguson FC Jr., Thiersch JB, Philips FS. The action of 4-amino-N10-methyl-pteroylglutamic acid in mice, rats and dogs. J Pharmacol Exp Ther 1950; 98: 293-9

11. Bruce WR, Meeker BE, Valeriote FA. Comparison of the sensivity of normal hematopoetic and transplanted lymphoma colonyforming cells to chemotherapeutic agents administered in vivo. J Natl Cancer Inst 1966; 37: 233-45

12. Roenigk HH, Haserick JR, Curtis GH. Methotrexate for psoriasis. A preliminary report. Cleve Clin Q 1965; 32: 211-15

13. Weinstein GD, Frost P. Methotrexate for psoriasis. Arch Derm 1971; 103: 33-8

14. Black RL, O`Brien WM, van Scott EJ, Auerbach R, Eisen AZ, Bunim JJ. Methotrexate therapy in psoriatic arthritis. Double-blind study in 21 patients. JAMA 1964; 180: 141-5

15. Spiegelberg HL, Miescher PA. The effect of 6-mercaptopurine and methotrexate on experimental immune thyroiditis in guinea pigs. J Exp Med 1963; 118: 869

16. Miescher PA, Riethmuller D. Diagnosis and treatment of systemic lupus erythematosus. Semin Haematol 1965; 2:1

17. Gross D, Enderlin M, Fehr K. Die immunsuppressive Behandlung der progredient chronischen Polyarthritis mit Antimetabolica und Cytostatika. Schweiz Med Wschr 1967; 97: 1301

18. Hoffmeister RT. Methotrexate in rheumatoid arthritis (abstract). Arthritis Rheum 1972;15: 114

19. Hoffmeister RT. Methotrexate therapy in Rheumatoid arthritis: 15 years experience. Am J Med 1983; 75 (6A): 69-73

20. Wilke WS, Calabrese LH, Scherbel AL. Methotrexate in the treatment of rheumatoid arthritis. Pilot study. Cleve Clin Q 1980; 47: 305-9

21. Willkens RF, et al. Low-dose pulse methotrexate in rheumatoid arthritis. J Rheumatol 1980; 7: 501-5

22. Willkens RF, Watson MA. Methotrexate: A perspektive of its use in the tratment of rheumatic disease. J Lab Clin Med 1982; 100: 314-21

23. Karger T, Rau R. Methotrexat-Behandlung hochaktiver chronischer Polyarthritiden. Münch Med Wschr 1984; 126: 560

24. Karger T, Rau R. Methotrexate therapy ofhighly active polyarthritis. Rheumatology 1986; 9: 154

25. Weinstein A, Marlowe S, Korn J, Farouhar F. Effect of methotrexate on rheumatoid arthritis: A systematic analysis of 21 patients. Rheumatology 1986; 9: 148

26. Williams HJ, et al. Comparison of low-dose oral pulse methotrexate and placebo in the treatment of rheumatoid arthritis. A controlled clinical trial. Arthr Rheum 1985; 28: 721-30

27. Williams HJ, et al. Methotrexate and placebo therapy in rheumatoid arthritis. Rheumatology 1986; 9: 174

28. Weinblatt ME, Coblyn JS, Fox DA, et al. Efficacy of low-dose methotrexate in rheumatoid arthritis. N Engl J Med 1985; 312: 818-22

29. Andersen PA, West SG, O`Dell JR et al. Weekly pulse methotrexate in rheumatoid arthritis. Ann Intern Med 1985; 103: 489-96

30. Thompson RN, Watts C, Edelman J, Russell AS. A controlled two-centre trial of parenteral methotrexate therapy for refractory rheumatoid arthritis. J Rheumatol 1984; 11: 760-2

31. Tugwell P, Bennett K, Gent M. Methotrexate in rheumatoid arthritis. Ann Intern Med 1987; 107: 358-66

32. Furst DE, Koehnke R, Burmeister LF, et al. Increasing methotrexate effect with increasing dose in the treatment of resistant rheumatoid arthritis. J Rheumatol 1989; 16: 313-20

33. Russell AS, Watts C, Thompson R, Edelman J, EsdaileJ, Percy J, et al. A double-blind placebo controlled short-term trial of parenteral methotrexate in rheumatoid arthritis. Arthritis Rheum 1984; 27: S59 (abstract)

34. Rau R, Herborn G. Intravenous treatment of highly active rheumatoid arthritis with methotrexate. In: Rau R (ed) Low dose methotrexate therapy in rheumatic diseases. Karger, Basel 1986

35. Michaels RM, Nashel DJ, Leonard A, Sliwinski J, Derbes SJ. Weekly intravenous methotrexate in the treatment of rheumatoid arthritis. Arthritis Rheum 1982; 25: 339-341

36. Weinblatt ME, Kaplan H,Germain BF. Low-dose methotrexate compared with auranofin in adult rheumatoid arthritis. Arthritis Rheum 1990; 33: 330-8

37. Williams HJ, Ward JR, Reading JC, et al: Comparison of auranofin, methotrxate, and the combination of both in the treatment of rheumatoid arthritis. Arthritis Rheum 1992; 3: 259-69

38. Morrasut T, Goldstein R, Cyr M, et al: Goldsodiumthiomalat compared to low-dose methotrexate in the treatment of rheumatoid arthritis - a randomised double-blind 26-week trial. J Rheumatol 1989; 16: 302-6

39. Suarez-Almazor ME, Fitzgerald A, Grace M, Russell AS: A randomised controlled trial of parenteral methotrexate compared with sodium aurothiomalate J Rheumatol 1988; 15: 753-56

40. Rau R, Herborn G, Karger T, et al A double blind randomised parallel trial of intramuscular methotrexate and goldsodiumthiomalate in early erosive rheumatoid arthritis. J Rheumatol 1991 18: 328-33

41. Rau R, Herborn G, Menninger H, Blechschmidt J: Comparison of intramuscular methotrexate and gold sodium thiomalate in the treatment of early erosive rheumatoid arthritis: 12 month data of a double-blind parallel study of 174 patients. Brit J Rheum 1997; 36: 345-52

42. Menninger H, Herborn G, Blechschmidt J, Rau R: A 36-month comparative trial of methotrexate and gold sodium thiomalate in the treatment of early active and erosive rheumatoid arthritis. Brit J Rheum 1998 37: 1060-1068

43. Sander O, Herborn G, Bock E, Rau R: Prospective six year follow up of patients withdrawn from a randomised study comparing parenteral gold salt and methotrexate. Ann Rheum Dis 1999; 58: 281-7

44. Hamdy H, McKendry RJR, Mierins E, Liver JA: Low-dose methotrexate compared with azathioprine in the treatment of rheumatoid arthritis. Arthritis Rheum 1987; 30: 361-8

45. Jeurissen MEC,Boerbooms AMTh, van de Putte et al : Methotrexate versus azathioprine in the treatment of rheumatoid arthritis. A forty- eight-week randomised, double blind trial. Arthritis Rheum 1991; 34: 951-60

46. Felson DT, Anderson JJ, Meenan RF: The comparative efficacy and toxicity of second-line drugs in rheumatoid arthritis. Arthrits Rheum 1990; 33: 1449-60

47. Nyfors A. Liver biopsies from psoriatics related to methotrexate therapy. Acta Pathol Microbiol 1977; 85: 511-8

48. Dahl MGC, Gregory MM, Scheuer PJ: Methotrexate hepatotoxicity in psoriasis – comparison of different dose regimes. Br Med J 1972; i: 654-6

49. Rau R, Karger T, Herborn G, Frenzel H. Liver biopsy findings in patients with rheumatoid arthritis under going long-term treatment with methotrexate. J Rheumatol 1989; 16: 489-93

50. Kremer JM. Liver biopsies in patients with rheumatoid arthritis receiving methotrexate: Where are we going? J Rheumatol 1992; 19: 189-91

51. Aponte J, Petrelli M. Histopathologic findings in the liver of rheumatoid arthritis patients treated with longterm bolus methotrexate. Arthritis Rheum1988; 31: 1457-64

52. Kremer JM, Phelps CT. Long-term prospective study of the use of methotrexate in the treatment of rheumatoid arthritis. Arthritis Rheum 1992; 35: 138-145

53. Rau R, Schleusser B, Herborn G, Karger T. Long-term treatment of destructive rheumatoid arthritis with methotrexate. J Rheumatol 1997; 24: 1881-89

54. Ortiz Z, Suarez Almazor M, Moher D, Wells G, Tugwell P. Folic acid and folinic acid for reducing side effects in patients receiving methotrexate for rheumatoid arthritis. Cochrane Database Syst Rev 2000; 2: CD00951

55. Braun J, Kästner P, Flaxenberg P et al. MC-MTX.6/ RH Study Group. Comparison of the clinical efficacy and safety of subcutaneous versus oral administration of methotrexate in patients with active rheumatoid arthritis. Results of a six-month, multicenter, randomized, double-blind, controlled, phase IV trial. Arthritis Rheum 2008; 58: 73-81

56. Klareskog L, van der Heijde D, de Jager JP, Gough A, Kalden J, Malaise M, Martin Mola E, Pavelka K, Sany J, Settas L, Wajdula J, Pedersen R, Fatenejad S, Sanda M; TEMPO (Trial of Etanercept and Methotrexate with Radiographic Patient Outcomes) study investigators. Therapeutic effect of the combination of etanercept and methotrexate compared with each treatment alone in patients with rheumatoid arthritis: double-blind randomised controlled trial. Lancet 2004; 363: 675-81

57. Breedveld FC, Weisman MH, Kavanaugh AF et al. A multicenter, randomized, double-blind clinical trial of combination therapy with adalimumab plus methotrexate versus methotrexate alone or adalimumab alone in patients with early, aggressive rheumatoid arthritis who had not had previous methotrexate treatment. Arthritis Rheum 2006; 54: 26-37

58. Maini R, William St, Clair E, Breedveld F, Furst D, Kalden J, et al. for the ATTRACT Study group. Infliximab versus placebo in rheumatoid arthritis patients receiving concomitant methotrexate: a randomised phase III trial. Lancet 1999; 354: 1932-39

59. Pincus T, Yazici Y, Sokka T, Aletaha D, Smolen JS. Methotrexate as the "anchor drug" for the treatment of early rheumatoid arthritis. Clin Exp Rheumatol 2003; 21 (Suppl. 31): 179-S185.

60. Smolen JS et al. EULAR recommendations for the management of rheumatoid arthritis with synthetic and biological disease modifying drugs: 2013 update. Ann Rheum Dis 2014; 73: 492-509

61. Krüger K et al. S1-Leitlinie zur sequentiellen medikamentösen Therapie der Rheumatoiden Arthritis 2012 Z Rheumatol 2012; 71: 592-603

62. Rau R, Methotrexat. Z Rheumatol 2016; 75: 599-603

63. Smolen JS, Landewé RBM, Bergstra SA, Kerschbaumer A, Sepriano A, Aletaha D, Caporali R, Edwards CJ, Hyrich KL, Pope JE, de Souza S, Stamm TA, Takeuchi T, Verschueren P, Winthrop KL, Balsa A, Bathon JM, Buch MH, Burmester GR, Buttgereit F, Cardiel MH, Chatzidionysiou K, Codreanu C, Cutolo M, den Broeder AA, El Aoufy K, Finckh A, Fonseca JE, Gottenberg JE, Haavardsholm EA, Iagnocco A, Lauper K, Li Z, McInnes IB, Mysler EF, Nash P, Poor G, Ristic GG, Rivellese F, Rubbert-Roth A, Schulze-Koops H, Stoilov N, Strangfeld A,

van der Helm-van Mil A, van Duuren E, Vliet Vlieland TPM, Westhovens R, van der Heijde D. EULAR recommendations for the management of rheumatoid arthritis with synthetic and biological disease-modifying antirheumatic drugs: 2022 update. Ann Rheum Dis 2023; 82(1): 3-18

65. Fiehn C, Krüger K. Therapiealgorithmus der rheumatoiden Arthritis. Z Rheumatol 2019; 78: 529-539

2. Pharmacology of methotrexate

2.1. Structure

Methotrexate (MTX) – 2-4-diamino-N10-methyl-pteroyl-glutamic acid – is a folic acid analogue which differs from folic acid (pteroylglutamic acid) by an amino substitution for hydroxyl at position 4 and a methyl group instead of hydrogen at position 10 (☞ Figure 2.1).

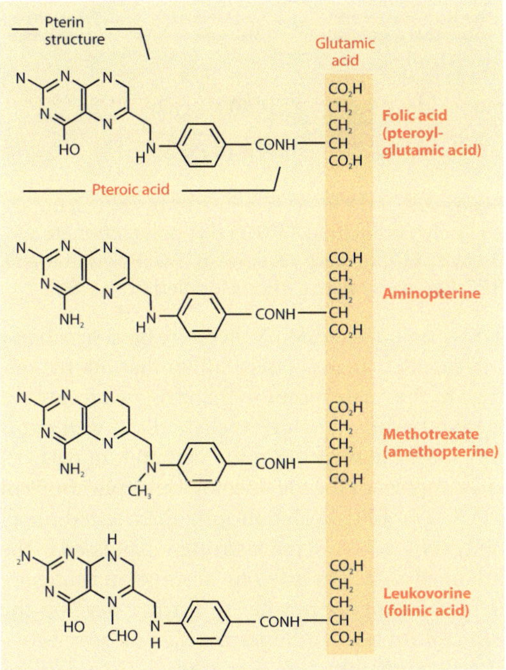

Figure 2.1: Comparison of the structure of folic acid, aminopterin, methotrexate and leucovorin (folinic acid).

2.2. Absorption and route of administration

The mechanism of absorption of MTX after oral administration was surprisingly only deciphered until 2006 (1). MTX is predominantly absorbed by the proton-coupled folate transporter (PCFT) in the proximal small intestine (2). This transporter, through which humans physiologically absorb folate, is active in an acidic environment and has an optimum pH of 5.5. Absorption is competitively inhibited by folates simultaneously present in the diet. Folate deficiency leads to an upregulation of PCFT, while alcohol consumption downregulates it. The absorption of oral MTX can therefore be influenced by a whole range of factors, including altered pH in the small intestine, e.g. through the use of proton pump inhibitors, but also the dietary ingestion of folates or alcohol. A second, quantitatively much less important absorption pathway of MTX is the reduced folate carrier (RFC), which is ubiquitously present on all body cells and has a pH optimum of >7. In patients with a hereditary defect in PCFT, it has been shown that this pathway is barely sufficient for absorbing the vital amounts of folate (2). With an oral dose of 15 mg, the area under the curve (AUC) of the absorbed MTX reaches a plateau (☞ Figure 2.2), meaning that even a further increase in the dose cannot increase the AUC (3). However, MTX bioavailability can be increased by 28% by splitting the dose (4).

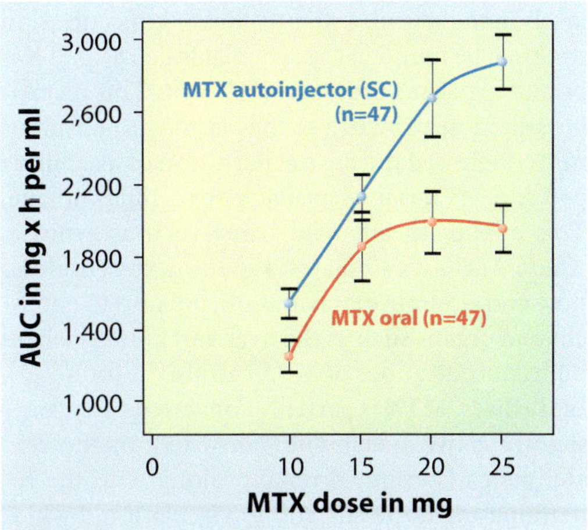

Figure 2.2: The absorption of orally administered MTX (**red**), but not of subcutaneously administered MTX (**blue**), reaches a plateau at around 15 mg, measured by the area under the curve (AUC) of MTX in plasma. Modified from (3).

The bioavailability of oral administration is variable because of the many factors influencing absorption. It was shown early on that it can fluctuate between 28 and 94% for oral administration (5).

Parenteral administration, which does not reach a plateau even when the dose is increased above 15 mg, therefore has considerable advantages over oral administration. For reasons of practicality, parenteral administration is now only applied subcutaneously (SC), and no longer intramuscularly or intravenously (6).

Braun et al. were able to show that MTX administered SC is approximately 40% more effective than oral MTX at the same dose (7). Parenteral MTX also induces the formation of polyglutamates of MTX, the active intracellular metabolite, more strongly than oral MTX.

2.3. Pharmacokinetics and metabolization

After oral administration, MTX floods into the peripheral blood after just over an hour and reaches a maximum concentration of 0.31 to 0.72 µmol/l at a dose of 15 mg. After initially higher levels in the serum, a slightly higher concentration can then be found in the synovial fluid (8). MTX is bound to plasma proteins by 42-57%. This reversible adhesion, primarily to the plasma protein albumin, is released during the perfusion of a capillary bed and MTX is then available for cellular uptake. This applies to inflamed tissue such as synovia, where MTX accumulates due to increased blood flow and albumin extravasation, but also to parenchymal organs such as the liver and kidney, where high concentrations of MTX can also be found (9). In the liver, MTX is partially converted to the only slightly active metabolite 7-hydroxy-methotrexate, which is excreted renally, along with the remaining methotrexate still in circulation, by glomerular filtration and tubular secretion with a half-life of 2 to 4 hours. 9-26% of MTX is excreted hepatobiliarily. Enterohepatic recirculation of this portion and MTX portions mobilized from compartments and tissues results in a second half-life of 15 to 21 hours. Overall, the plasma half-life of MTX is given as 6 to 7 hours and the renal clearance as an average of 110 ml/min. In renal insufficiency, MTX accumulates strongly because excretion is delayed.

MTX only becomes effective after intracellular uptake in the target tissue (☞ Figure 2.3). This occurs both via folate receptors and via the RFC (10). Among the folate receptors, folate receptor β plays a particularly important role, as it is expressed on differentiated myelomonocytic cells, activated monocytes/macrophages and neutrophil granulocytes. It is detected on synovial macrophages in the inflammatory tissue of arthritis, where it is upregulated to meet the folic acid requirement during inflammation (11).

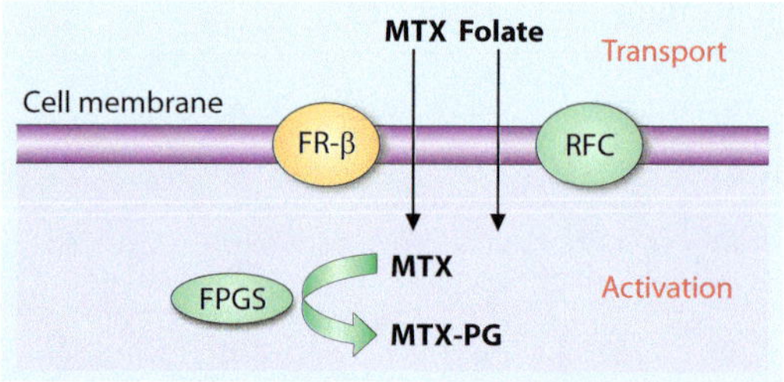

Figure 2.3: MTX effect is regulated by cellular uptake and polyglutamation. **FPGS**: Folyl-polyglutamate synthetase, **FR-**β: Folate receptor-β, **PG**: Polyglutamate, **RFC**: Reduced folate carrier. Modified from (18).

To a certain degree, MTX therefore has a selectively increased effect in synovial inflammation. In contrast to the folate receptor-β, the folate receptor-α is found primarily on epithelial cells as well as tumors. This absorption route is therefore particularly important for the oncological applications of MTX. The RFC is ubiquitously distributed on all body cells and is not more strongly expressed in the inflamed joint. The different absorption routes are the subject of approaches to further develop the principle of folate inhibition with a more selective effect on inflammation. For example, folate receptor-β-specific folate inhibitors are being developed, which are said to have a better effect and lower toxicity, particularly due to a lack of affinity for the RFC (9).

After intracellular uptake, an activation step takes place. The enzyme folyl-polyglutamate synthetase (FPGS) binds up to 5 glutamate residues to MTX (12). Since MTX in the polyglutamated form can no longer leave the cell, polyglutamation extends the intracellular half-life. In addition, polyglutamation gives MTX a higher folate-inhibitory effect. Polyglutamated MTX, especially the metabolites with a high number of glutamates, is therefore the actual active metabolite of MTX. Gamma-glutamate hydrolase finally splits off the glutamates so that MTX can leave the cell and be excreted. The kinetics of the formation of the polyglutamated MTX metabolites after MTX has been administered and their degradation after treatment has ended (☞ Figure 2.4a+b) correlate well with the slow onset of the clinical effect and its decline. For methodological reasons, the polyglutamated MTX metabolites are measured in erythrocytes. However, the enzymes for polyglutamation can also be detected in the synovia, so it can be assumed that polyglutamation also takes place in the same form in the inflammatory synovia.

The rate of polyglutamation, like other enzyme activities, is subject to very large inter-individual fluctuations of up to a factor 40 (13). Various other factors can also influence the rate of polyglutamation measured in erythrocytes. For example, a higher rate of polyglutamated MTX is formed with parenteral compared to oral MTX therapy (14). Smoking and concomitant therapy with NSAIDs, on the other hand, reduce polyglutamation. From cross-sectional studies, it was difficult to determine whether the response to MTX is actually associated with the rate of polyglutamation of MTX. However, two prospective studies show a clear correlation between polyglutamated MTX metabolites and response to disease activity in both JIA (15) and RA (16). In JIA, however, only the long-chain forms with three or more glutamate tails were clearly associated. In RA, a cut-off value of 74 nmol/l of the total number of polyglutamated MTX molecules was found for response. In both entities, no association between the amount of polyglutamated MTX metabolites and toxicity was found.

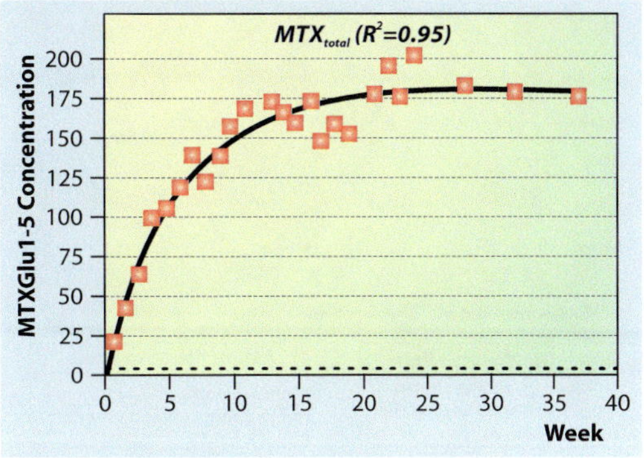

a

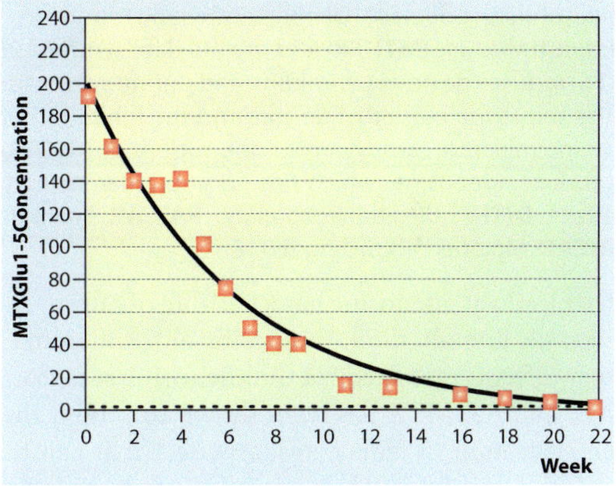

b

Figures 2.4a+b: Pharmacokinetics of MTX polyglutamates, the active intracellular metabolites of MTX, in erythrocytes after initiation (**a**) and after discontinuation (**b**) of MTX therapy. Modified from (12).

2.4. Mechanism of action

Although MTX inhibits folate-dependent enzymes as an antimetabolite, the antiproliferative and immunosuppressive effect of MTX is considered to be low in the small doses used in rheumatology. This is supported by the fact that MTX plays no role as an immunosuppressant in organ transplants and no increased rate of opportunistic infections was found in RA patients due to MTX in large registers.

MTX, on the other hand, has strong immunomodulatory and anti-inflammatory effects. The induction of extracellular adenosine, which is induced via the inhibition of AICAR transformylase and subsequently via several metabolic pathways, appears to play an important role (☞ Figure 2.5).

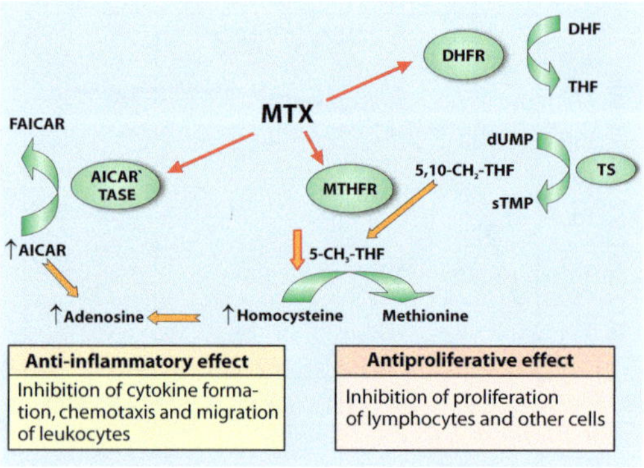

Figure 2.5: MTX blocks folic acid-dependent enzymes and induces adenosine. The inhibition of dihydrofolate reductase (**DHFR**), methylene tetrahydrofolate reductase (**MTHFR**) and thymidylate synthetase (**TS**) reduces de novo pyrimidine and purine synthesis. The reduction of methyl donors and the inhibition of aminoimidazole carboxyamido ribonucleotide (**AICAR**) produce adenosine, which has an anti-inflammatory effect. **D/TH**F: di/tetrahydrofolate, **FAICAR**: **formyl-AICAR**. Modified according to (18).

Extracellular adenosine has a half-life of only a few seconds in body fluid. Its specific anti-inflammatory effect is mediated via the adenosine receptors A2a and A3. MTX has been shown to inhibit the extravasation of leukocytes, an effect that can be specifically inhibited by adenosine receptor blockade (17, 18). Further multiple biological effects of MTX in the target tissue are listed in Table 2.1. Overall, MTX inhibits important cellular and humoral inflammatory mechanisms that play a role in the maintenance of arthritis, but also other forms of autoimmune inflammation in tissue (18). It is likely that MTX has a significant effect on the cellular compartment of monocytes and macrophages and their extravasation, cellular activity and production of inflammatory mediators. This is also mediated by the increased expression of folate receptor-β described above and thus the likely preferential uptake of MTX by these cells during inflammation.

MTX has a significant cardioprotective effect in RA and reduces the risk of a cardiovascular event in a patient with RA by half after 22-40 months and even by over 80% in the further course (19).

In RA patients who respond to MTX therapy, mortality is also significantly reduced in the long term (20). There is evidence that not only the suppression of inflammation, but possibly an independent effect on mortality exist , such as a direct therapeutic effect on the development of arteriosclerosis (21). This theory is supported by the fact that MTX inhibits the formation of foam cell macrophages by activating reverse cholesterol transport (22). This effect is also mediated via the adenosine receptor. The idea that these effects are based on specific effects on arteriosclerosis and not just a general control of inflammation is also supported by the fact that previous studies could not demonstrate positive effects on the reduction of mortality when using parenteral gold (23), despite its recognized good effect on disease activity. However, the prospective randomized CIRT study in patients with stable arteriosclerosis was unable to show a reduction in the number of cardiovascular events through MTX therapy (24).

Adenosine-specific effects may also be responsible for adverse effects of MTX: For example, *in vitro*, MTX induces the formation of giant cells by cultured monocytes in an adenosine receptor-dependent manner (25), an effect that could possibly explain the increased occurrence of rheumatoid nodules during MTX therapy. Binding of adenosine receptors in the CNS can also trigger fatigue (26) and fibrosis of the liver (27). Both are possible adverse effects of MTX, but cases of liver fibrosis are very rare.

Summary of MTX Pharmacology	
Approved indications (except malignant diseases)	• Active rheumatoid arthritis • Severe, active juvenile idiopathic arthritis • Severe psoriasis vulgaris • Psoriatic arthritis
Active metabolites	MTX polyglutamate (intracellular)
Mechanism of action	• Inhibition of dihydrofolate reductase and other folate-dependent enzymes • Induction of adenosine by inhibition of 5-aminoimidazole-4-carboxamide ribonucleotide (AICAR) transformylase
Effect on target cells (at low doses)	• Inhibition of migration and chemotaxis of neutrophil granulocytes and the production of proinflammatory cytokines • Promotion of apoptosis of monocytic cells through a JUN kinase-dependent mechanism • Inhibition of cartilage invasion by synovial fibroblasts and macrophage function • Inhibition of the production of metalloproteinases, collagenases, prostaglandin E2 and superoxide
Plasma half time	5 to 8 hours (intracellular persistance of metabolites for weeks)
Elimination	Predominantly renal elimination
Dosage and mode of application	15-25 mg once a week orally or subcutaneously
Recommended comedication	Folate 5-15 mg orally 24-48 hours after MTX application
Most important adverse effects (at low doses)	Increase in transaminases, nausea, dizziness, stomatitis, cytopenia, rarely allergic-toxic pneumonitis, teratogenicity
Follow-ups	Without further risk factors, check blood count, GPT/ALT, GOT/AST, γ-GT and creatinine (with calculated GFR) • at initiation of treatment (baseline) • then weeks 2, 4 and 6 • then every 1-3 months

Tab. 2.1: Summary of key data on MTX.

2.5. Folic acid supplementation

To reduce the undesirable effects of MTX therapy, the administration of folic acid at a dose of 5(-15) mg per week 24 hours after MTX administration is recommended (28).

A Cochrane meta-analysis comes to the conclusion that supplementation of both folic acid and the more expensive folinic acid significantly reduce gastrointestinal side effects and transaminase increases when using MTX (29). In addition, folic acid supplementation reduces the rate of discontinuation of MTX therapy. In contrast, in this meta-analysis, the evidence for a weakening of the therapeutic effect of MTX is assessed as unclear, although there were earlier data analyses of clinical studies that indicated a weakening of the MTX effect through folate supplementation (30). The dose of 5 mg once a week 24 hours after MTX recommended by the professional association was chosen empirically. A recent study comparing doses of 10 and 30 mg of folate per week could not show a benefit from the higher dose (31). The action of MTX via the non-folate-dependent adenosine pathway described above explains this presumed discrepancy in the effect of folic acid on adverse effects and its therapeutic effect.

2.6. Methotrexate effect as a combination partner with biologics

MTX is also important as a combination partner. It has been shown that the effect of TNF-α inhibitors and the anti-CD20 antibody rituximab is improved when combined with MTX.

In addition to a synergistic effect of MTX with the respective biologic, the inhibition of the formation of antibodies directed against them (human anti-drug antibodies = HADA) is crucial. Such HADA can have a neutralizing effect and shorten the half-life of the drugs. For the TNF-α inhibitors infliximab (INX), golimumab and adalimumab (ADA), the inhibition of HADA formation by MTX has been reliably demonstrated. In the case of ADA, HADA was detectable in 12% of patients with MTX therapy, compared to 38% without MTX (32). Interestingly, polyglutamation as an activation step of MTX again appears to be of crucial importance. Dervieux et al. were able to demonstrate that patients who received MTX and INX in combination developed antibodies against INX significantly less frequently and showed higher INX concentrations in the serum when the concentrations of at least triply polyglutamated MTX were above 50 pmol/l (33). Surprisingly, relatively low doses of MTX are sufficient to cause the suppressive effect of MTX on HADA formation. In the CONCERTO study, 10 mg orally once per week was just as effective as 20 mg per week in achieving the effect of suppressing HADA formation and thus an enhanced effect of ADA therapy given in combination (34). This was not due to incomplete absorption of oral MTX therapy at higher doses, since significantly higher concentrations of polyglutamated MTX were detected in the erythrocytes at a dose of 20 mg MTX per week, without this resulting in an increased effect (35). While MTX doses of at least 15 mg per week were found to be optimal doses in prospective dose-finding studies for MTX monotherapy, a lower dose seems likely to be sufficient in combination with a biologic. However, this should be confirmed in further studies with a more representative patient population than the MTX-naive population of the CONCERTO study.

2.7. Genetic markers as predictors of methotrexate effect

A large number of genetic markers, which affect genes of folic acid metabolism, transport and activation of MTX and adenosine formation and effect, have been described as markers mainly for toxicity, but less frequently also for the effectivity of MTX. Wessels et al. (36) have proposed a composite clinical and pharmacogenetic score that includes the parameters

- female gender
- DAS28 before therapy >3.8
- smoking status and
- RF positivity

as clinical parameters and the genotypes *MTHFD1 1958AA*, *AMPD1 34CC*, *ITPA 94A* and *ATIC 347G* in a point scale. According to the authors, this score allows a prediction for 60% of patients, whereas this is only the case for 35% of patients using clinical criteria alone without genetic markers. In these patients, there is a 95% certainty that they will respond, or in the other case there is a 86% certainty that they will not respond. However, this score has not yet been used in clinical practice. The development of practical genetic markers that predict the response or toxicity of MTX is made difficult by the fact that the significance and predictive value of various genetic predictors is generally low and the results are often not equally reproducible in different populations, meaning that meta-analyses of the data produce different results. The score has not been adopted in practice.

2.8. Interactions

Interactions are the most common reason for MTX-induced pancytopenia, which has a high mortality rate (37). The simultaneous administration of cotrimoxazole as an antibiotic in a therapeutic dose of usually 2 × 960 mg per day is probably the most dangerous combination (38). There are a large number of case reports in the literature, often with fatal outcomes, so it is strictly contraindicated. It is important, however, that the administration of 960 mg cotrimoxazole 3 × weekly as *Pneumocystis jirovecii* prophylaxis does not trigger any corresponding toxicities. A case-control study was able to show that the risk of cytopenias from the combination of MTX and cotrimoxazole is not increased at this low prophylactic dose (39).

The situation is similar with the administration of acetylsalicylic acid (ASA) in analgesic doses of 2 g or more, which also have a high risk of interaction with MTX (40). However, ASA is rarely used in Rheumatology these days. The frequently given dose of 80-100 mg/day ASA for platelet aggregation inhibition has no clinically relevant interactions with MTX and can be safely given as a co-medication with MTX.

The combination of MTX with non-steroidal antirheumatic drugs (NSAIDs) (40) has also been correlated with cytopenias. However, direct pharmacodynamic interactions between NSAIDs, including modern coxibs, and MTX were not found (41-43), so the explanation probably lies primarily in the potential impairment of renal function by NSAIDs.

The combination of MTX with the antibiotic isoniazide for the treatment of latent tuberculosis and the DMARD leflunomide (LEF) can lead to increases in transaminases (44, 45). Cytopenias have also been described in the case of LEF (46). Both drugs play an important role in the guideline-based management of RA when combined with MTX, and dangerous findings from interactions are rare. There is also a current large registry evaluation for the combination of MTX and LEF, which demonstrates the general safety (47).

With regular monitoring of the relevant laboratory parameters, the combinations of LEF or isoniazide with MTX are therefore justified.

The combination of MTX with the DMARD sulfasalazine (SSZ) and hydroxychloroquine (HCQ) has been proven as triple therapy for RA and, despite theoretical interactions between MTX and SSZ via folic acid levels, is also safe and adverse effects are rare (48).

Probenecide hardly plays a role in the treatment of gout anymore. Due to interference with tubular excretion and the resulting pancytopenia (49), it should not be given in combination with MTX.

It is somewhat unclear whether and to what extent MTX interacts with penicillins. However, the combination has been associated with pancytopenia (50), which can be explained by the competition between the two substances for plasma protein binding. Since antibiotic therapy is temporary and MTX can be paused for 2-3 weeks without loss of effectivity, it is recommended that MTX therapy should generally be interrupted when penicillin antibiotics are administered.

According to an analysis of the Eudra Vigilance database, the combination of MTX with metamizole can lead to a rate of agranulocytosis that is approximately 4.5 times higher, on average (51). The increased risk of this combination is evident from the age of 40 (OR 2.6), but is highest from the age of 80 (OR 8.1). The rate of fatal outcomes for this complication of combined therapy is 17% across all age groups. In this analysis, children and adolescents under 18 years of age had no increased risk of agranulocytosis when combining MTX and metamizole.

It should be mentioned that the combination of MTX with both biological (B) and targeted synthetic (ts) DMARDs (JAK inhibitors) has not shown any safety indications for interactions.

2.9. Dosage in elderly patients and in renal insufficiency

Various studies have shown that it is not age *per se*, but organ function and co-medications that determine the dose of MTX (52). The common adverse effect of nausea with MTX occurs more frequently in younger people than in older people (53). Since renal function can be unstable in old age, the author recommends considering gradually increasing the dose by 10 mg per week from the age of around 75 years, or generally not exceeding 10 mg per week over the age of 80 (☞ Table 2.2). However, the procedure depends heavily on the biological age of the patient.

Pharmacological studies show that from a glomerular filtration rate (GFR) of <45 ml/min, the plasma concentration and half-life of MTX increase significantly, while the changes are still small at a GFR of 45 to 60 ml/min (54). Accordingly, the author recommends a dose adjustment as shown in Table 2.3. Possible rapid changes in renal function due to changes in co-medication or concomitant diseases must be taken into account for the dosing decision.

Substance/ Substance class	Mechanisms of interaction (selection)	Possible consequences	Clinical significance	Ref.
Interactions with published evidence				
Acetylsalicylic acid (analgetic dosages >2 g per day)	Reduced tubular secretion, competition for plasma protein adhesion	Increase of effect and toxicity	A	37, 38
Acetylsalicylic acid (dosages for inhibition of thrombocyte aggregation at 80-100 mg per day)		None	D	–
Cotrimoxazole (therapeutic dosages of 2 × 960 mg per day)	Additive folate-antagonistic effect and bone marrow toxicity	Increase of effect and toxicity	A	37, 38
Cotrimoxazole (dosages for *Pneumocystis* prophylaxis 960 mg 3 × per week)		None	D	39
Isoniazide (for treatment of latent tuberculosis at 300 mg per day)	Additive hepatotoxicity	Elevated transaminases	C	44
Leflunomide (for combination treatment of RA with csDMARD at 10-20 mg per day)	Additive hepato- and hematotoxicity	Elevated transaminases and cytopenias	C	45-47
NSAIDs	Reduced tubular secretion, reduced kidney function, competition for plasma protein adhesion	Increase of effect and toxicity	C	40-43
Penicillins	Competition for plasma protein adhesion	Increase of effect and toxicity	B	50
Probenecide	Reduced renal elimination of MTX	Increase of effect and toxicity	B	49
Sulfasalazine	Inhibition of folic acid synthesis	Increase of effect and toxicity	D	48
Metamizole	Synergistic bone marrow toxicity	Increased rates of agranulocytosis	B (A for age ≥80 y)	51
Further interactions according to summary of product characteristics				
Protein-bound drugs like salicylates, hypoglycemic drugs, diuretics, sulfonamide, diphenylhydantoine, tetracyclines, chloramphenicol and p-aminobenzoic acid as well as acidic anti-inflammatory substances	Competition for plasma protein adhesion	Increase of effect and toxicity	A-C	–
Oral antibiotics like tetracyclines, chloramphenicol and non-absorbable broad spectrum antibiotics	Influence on enterohepatic circulation via changes in gut microbiome	Increase of effect and toxicity	C	–
Theophylline	Reduction of theophylline clearance	Increase of theophylline levels	C	–
Bone marrow toxic substances like azathioprine, chloramphenicol, mercaptopurine, pyrimethamine, retinoids, sulfonamide	Additive bone marrow toxicity and hematotoxicity	Pancytopenias and elevated transaminases	A-C	–
Renally active drugs like loop diuretics	Inhibition of renal elimination of MTX	Increase of effect and toxicity	C	–
Proton pump inhibitors	Delayed renal elimination of MTX	Increase of effect and toxicity	D	–

Table 2.2: Mechanisms and assessment of the pharmacological interactions of methotrexate. The clinical significance is assessed by an expert vote after taking into account a systematic literature search (Fiehn C. et al., 2024) according to the following criteria:

A: Dangerous combination
B: Avoid combination (DMARD break if possible)
C: Possible combination with increased need for monitoring and possible dose adjustment
D: Pharmacological interaction without relevance in standard DMARD dosages

Age			
<65 years	65-75 years	>75 years	>80 years
No limitation	No limitation	Depends on biologic age and comorbidities, reduced starting dose, consider incremental dose adjustments	Depends on biologic age and comorbidities, 10 mg per week starting dose, consider incremental dose adjustments
Kidney function			
GFR <30 ml/min	GFR 30-45 ml/min	GFR 45-60 ml/min	GFR >60 ml/min
Contraindicated	<10 mg per week, only exceed this dose in exceptional cases	10 mg per week starting dose, consider incremental dose adjustments	15-25 mg per week

Table 2.3: Dosage recommendation of MTX according to age and renal function. Recommendation by expert vote after taking into consideration a systematic literature search (54).

2.10. References

1. Qiu A, Jansen M, Sakaris A, Min SH, Chattopadhyay S, Tsai E et al. Identification of an intestinal folate transporter and the molecular basis for hereditary folate malabsorption. Cell 2006; 127(5):917-28.

2. Visentin M, Diop-Bove N, Zhao R, Goldman ID. The intestinal absorption of folates. Annu Rev Physiol 2014; 76:251-74.

3. Schiff MH, Jaffe JS, Freundlich B. Head-to-head, randomised, crossover study of oral versus subcutaneous methotrexate in patients with rheumatoid arthritis: drug-exposure limitations of oral methotrexate at doses >/=15 mg may be overcome with subcutaneous administration. Ann Rheum Dis 2014; 73(8):1549-51.

4. Hoekstra M, Haagsma C, Neef C, Proost J, Knuif A, van de Laar M. Splitting high-dose oral methotrexate improves bioavailability: a pharmacokinetic study in patients with rheumatoid arthritis. J Rheumatol 2006; 33(3):481-5.

5. Bannwarth B, Pehourcq F, Schaeverbeke T, Dehais J. Clinical pharmacokinetics of low-dose pulse methotrexate in rheumatoid arthritis. Clin Pharmacokinet 1996; 30(3):194-210.

6. Muller-Ladner U, Rockwitz K, Brandt-Jurgens J, Haux R, Kastner P, Braun J et al. Tolerability and patient/physician satisfaction with subcutaneously administered methotrexate provided in two formulations of different drug concentrations in patients with rheumatoid arthritis. Open Rheumatol J 2010; 4:15-22.

7. Braun J, Kastner P, Flaxenberg P, Wahrisch J, Hanke P, Demary W et al. Comparison of the clinical efficacy and safety of subcutaneous versus oral administration of methotrexate in patients with active rheumatoid arthritis: results of a six-month, multicenter, randomized, double-blind, controlled, phase IV trial. Arthritis Rheum 2008; 58(1):73-81.

8. Tishler M, Caspi D, Graff E, Segal R, Peretz H, Yaron M. Synovial and serum levels of methotrexate during methotrexate therapy of rheumatoid arthritis. Br J Rheumatol 1989; 28(5):422-3.

9. Fiehn C. Methotrexate transport mechanisms: the basis for targeted drug delivery and ss-folate-receptor-specific treatment. Clin Exp Rheumatol 2010; 28(5 Suppl 61):S40-S45.

10. Elnakat H, Ratnam M. Distribution, functionality and gene regulation of folate receptor isoforms: implications in targeted therapy. Adv Drug Deliv Rev 2004; 56(8):1067-84.

11. Nakashima-Matsushita N, Homma T, Yu S, Matsuda T, Sunahara N, Nakamura T et al. Selective expression of folate receptor beta and its possible role in methotrexate transport in synovial macrophages from patients with rheumatoid arthritis. Arthritis Rheum 1999; 42(8):1609-16.

12. Dalrymple JM, Stamp LK, O'Donnell JL, Chapman PT, Zhang M, Barclay ML. Pharmacokinetics of oral methotrexate in patients with rheumatoid arthritis. Arthritis Rheum 2008; 58(11):3299-308.

13. Stamp LK, O'Donnell JL, Chapman PT, Zhang M, Frampton C, James J et al. Determinants of red blood cell methotrexate polyglutamate concentrations in rheumatoid arthritis patients receiving long-term methotrexate treatment. Arthritis Rheum 2009; 60(8):2248-56.

14. Becker ML, van HL, Gaedigk R, Lasky A, Hoeltzel M, Stobaugh J et al. Analysis of intracellular methotrexate polyglutamates in patients with juvenile idiopathic arthritis: effect of route of administration on variability in intracellular metho-

trexate polyglutamate concentrations. Arthritis Rheum 2010; 62(6):1803-12.

15. Calasan MB, den BE, de Rotte MC, Vastert SJ, Kamphuis S, de JR et al. Methotrexate polyglutamates in erythrocytes are associated with lower disease activity in juvenile idiopathic arthritis patients. Ann Rheum Dis 2015; 74(2):402-7.

16. de Rotte MC, den BE, de Jong PH, Pluijm SM, Calasan MB, Weel AE et al. Methotrexate polyglutamates in erythrocytes are associated with lower disease activity in patients with rheumatoid arthritis. Ann Rheum Dis 2015; 74(2):408-14.

17. Cronstein BN, Eberle MA, Gruber HE, Levin RI. Methotrexate inhibits neutrophil function by stimulating adenosine release from connective tissue cells. Proc Natl Acad Sci U S A 1991; 88(6):2441-5.

18. Wessels JA, Huizinga TW, Guchelaar HJ. Recent insights in the pharmacological actions of methotrexate in the treatment of rheumatoid arthritis. Rheumatology 2008; 47(3): 249-55.

19. Bili A, Tang X, Pranesh S, Bozaite R, Morris SJ, Antohe JL et al. Tumor necrosis factor alpha inhibitor use and decreased risk for incident coronary events in rheumatoid arthritis. Arthritis Care Res 2014; 66(3): 355-63.

20. Krause D, Schleusser B, Herborn G, Rau R. Response to methotrexate treatment is associated with reduced mortality in patients with severe rheumatoid arthritis. Arthritis Rheum 2000; 43(1):14-21.

21. Krause D, Gabriel B, Herborn G, Braun J, Rau R. The positive influence of methotrexate on the mortality of patients with rheumatoid arthritis is partly independent of its effect on disease activity: results of a re-evaluation 18 years after baseline. Clin Exp Rheumatol 2014; 32(3): 395-400.

22. Reiss AB, Carsons SE, Anwar K, Rao S, Edelman SD, Zhang H et al. Atheroprotective effects of methotrexate on reverse cholesterol transport proteins and foam cell transformation in human THP-1 monocyte/macrophages. Arthritis Rheum 2008; 58(12):3675-83.

23. Pincus T, Brooks RH, Callahan LF. Prediction of long-term mortality in patients with rheumatoid arthritis according to simple questionnaire and joint count measures. Ann Intern Med 1994; 120(1):26-34.

24. Ridker PM, Everett BM, Pradhan A, MacFadyen JG, Solomon DH Zaharris E et al; CIRT Investigators. Low-dose methotrexate for the prevention of atherosclerotic events. N Engl J Med. 2019;380:752-62.

25. Merrill JT, Shen C, Schreibman D, Coffey D, Zakharenko O, Fisher R et al. Adenosine A1 receptor promotion of multinucleated giant cell formation by human monocytes: a mechanism for methotrexate-induced nodulosis in rheumatoid arthritis. Arthritis Rheum 1997; 40(7):1308-15.

26. Diaz-Munoz M, Hernandez-Munoz R, Suarez J, Vidrio S, Yaanez L, Aguilar-Roblero R et al. Correlation between blood adenosine metabolism and sleep in humans. Sleep Res Online 1999; 2(2):33-41.

27. Peng Z, Borea PA, Varani K, Wilder T, Yee H, Chiriboga L et al. Adenosine signaling contributes to ethanol-induced fatty liver in mice. J Clin Invest 2009; 119(3): 582-94.

28. Tarner I, Manger B, Fleck M, Gromnica-Ihle E, Keyßer G, Köhler L. Evidenzbasierte Empfehlungen einer nationalen Expertenrunde zum Einsatz von Methotrexat bei entzündlich-rheumatischen Erkrankungen. Akt Rheumatol 2009; 34(01):59-66.

29. Shea B, Swinden MV, Tanjong GE, Ortiz Z, Katchamart W, Rader T et al. Folic acid and folinic acid for reducing side effects in patients receiving methotrexate for rheumatoid arthritis. Cochrane Database Syst Rev 2013; 5:CD000951.

30. Khanna D, Park GS, Paulus HE, Simpson KM, Elashoff D, Cohen SB et al. Reduction of the efficacy of methotrexate by the use of folic acid: post hoc analysis from two randomized controlled studies. Arthritis Rheum 2005; 52(10):3030-8.

31. Dhir V, Sandhu A, Kaur J, Pinto B, Kumar P, Kaur P et al. Comparison of two different folic acid doses with methotrexate - a randomized controlled trial (FOLVARI Study). Arthritis Res Ther 2015; 17:156.

32. Bartelds GM, Wijbrandts CA, Nurmohamed MT, Stapel S, Lems WF, Aarden L et al. Clinical response to adalimumab: relationship to anti-adalimumab antibodies and serum adalimumab concentrations in rheumatoid arthritis. Ann Rheum Dis 2007; 66(7):921-6.

33. Dervieux T, Weinblatt ME, Kivitz A, Kremer JM. Methotrexate polyglutamation in relation to infliximab pharmacokinetics in rheumatoid arthritis. Ann Rheum Dis 2013; 72(6): 908-10.

34. Burmester GR, Kivitz AJ, Kupper H, Arulmani U, Florentinus S, Goss SL et al. Efficacy and safety of ascending methotrexate dose in combination with adalimumab: the randomised CONCERTO trial. Ann Rheum Dis 2015; 74(6):1037-44.

35. Burmester GR, Kivitz A, Kupper H, Arulmani U, Florentinus S, Goss SL et al. Response to H Zeidler's comments on the CONCERTO study. Ann Rheum Dis 2014; 73(8):e51.

36. Wessels JA, van der Kooij SM, le CS, Kievit W, Barerra P, Allaart CF et al. A clinical pharmacogenetic model to predict the efficacy of methotrexate monotherapy in recent-onset rheumatoid arthritis. Arthritis Rheum 2007; 56(6):1765-75.

37. Lim AY, Gaffney K, Scott DG. Methotrexate-induced pancytopenia: serious and under-reported? Our experience of 25 cases in 5 years. Rheumatology (Oxford). 2005;44(8):1051-5.

38. Bourré-Tessier J, Haraoui B. Methotrexate drug interactions in the treatment of rheumatoid arthritis: a systematic review. J Rheumatol. 2010;37(7):1416-21.

39. Kwon OC, Lee JS, Kim YG et al. Safety of the concomitant use of methotrexate and a prophylactic dose of trimethoprim-sulfamethoxazole. Clin Rheumatol. 2018;37(12): 3215-3220.

40. Svanström H, Lund M, Melbye M, Pasternak B. Concomitant use of low-dose methotrexate and NSAIDs and the risk of serious adverse events among patients with rheumatoid arthritis. Pharmacoepidemiol Drug Saf. 2018;27(8):885-893.

41. Ahern M, Booth J, Loxton A et al. Methotrexate kinetics in rheumatoid arthritis: is there an interaction with nonsteroidal antiinflammatory drugs? J Rheumatol. 1988;15(9): 1356-60.

42. Schwartz JI, Agrawal NG, Wong PH et al. Examination of the effect of increasing doses of etoricoxib on oral methotrexate pharmacokinetics in patients with rheumatoid arthritis. J Clin Pharmacol. 2009;49(10):1202-9.

43. Karim A, Tolbert DS, Hunt TL et al. Celecoxib, a specific COX-2 inhibitor, has no significant effect on methotrexate pharmacokinetics in patients with rheumatoid arthritis. J Rheumatol. 1999;(12):2539-43

44. Vanhoof J, Landewe S, Van Wijngaerden E, Geusens P. High incidence of hepatotoxicity of isoniazid treatment for tuberculosis chemoprophylaxis in patients with rheumatoid arthritis treated with methotrexate or sulfasalazine and anti-tumour necrosis factor inhibitors. Ann Rheum Dis. 2003; 62(12):1241-2.

45. Bird P, Griffiths H, Tymms K et al. The SMILE study — safety of methotrexate in combination with leflunomide in rheumatoid arthritis. J Rheumatol. 2013;40(3):228-35.

46. Chan J, Sanders DC, Du L, Pillans PI. Leflunomide-associated pancytopenia with or without methotrexate. Ann Pharmacother. 2004;38(7-8):1206-11.

47. Bredemeier M, Ranza R, Kakehasi AM et al. Safety of the methotrexate-leflunomide combination in rheumatoid arthritis: Results of a multicentric, registry-based, cohort study (Biobada Brasil). J Rheumatol. 20214;8(10):1519-1527.

48. Quach LT, Chang BH, Brophy MT et al. Rheumatoid arthritis triple therapy compared with etanercept: difference in infectious and gastrointestinal adverse events. Rheumatology (Oxford). 2017;56(3):378-383.

49. Basin KS, Escalante A, Beardmore TD. Severe pancytopenia in a patient taking low dose methotrexate and probenecid. J Rheumatol. 1991;18(4):609-10

50. Sathi N, Ackah J, Dawson J. Methotrexate induced neutropenia associated with coprescription of penicillins: serious and under-reported? Rheumatology (Oxford). 2006;45(3): 361-2

51. Homann F, Bantel C, Jobski K. Agranulocytosis attributed to metamizole: An analysis of spontaneous reports in EudraVigilance 1985-2017. Basic Clin Pharmacol Toxicol. 2019; 126:116-125

52. Bologna C, Viu P, Jorgensen C et al. Effect of age on the efficacy and tolerance of methotrexate in rheumatoid arthritis. Br J Rheumatol. 1996;35(5):453-7.

53. Patil P, Parker RA, Rawcliffe C et al. Methotrexate-induced nausea and vomiting in adolescent and young adult patients. Clin Rheumatol. 2014;33(3):403-7.

54. Bressolle F, Bologna C, Kinowski JM. Effects of moderate renal insufficiency on pharmacokinetics of methotrexate in rheumatoid arthritis patients. Ann Rheum Dis 1989;57:110-113

55. Fiehn C, Leipe J, Weseloh C, Bergner R, Krüger K. Assessment of interactions and dosage recommendations of synthetic DMARDs-Evidence-based and consensus-based recommendations based on a systematic literature search. Z Rheumatol. 2024 Feb;83(Suppl 1):8-19

3. Methotrexate monotherapy in rheumatoid arthritis

3.1. Effectivity in long-term studies

3.1.1. Long-term observational studies

After placebo-controlled studies were able to demonstrate the effectivity of methotrexate (MTX), the long-term tolerability and adverse event rate in long-term therapy became the subject of the first observational studies (☞ Table 3.1). It must be taken into account that, initially, the participants had almost exclusively been poor responders to conventional DMARDs such as gold, D-penicillamine, resochin or cytostatics like cyclophosphamide. Several studies consistently showed sustained clinical effectivity with a reduction in the number of swollen joints and a decrease in inflammatory parameters with a simultaneous reduction in the glucocorticoid (GC) dose. As the treating physicians became more confident in using MTX, the 5-year retention rate of MTX also increased from 39% to 64% of those treated. In a prospective study from Australia only 7% of study participants stopped taking MTX due to ineffectivity (1). This made MTX the DMARD with the highest retention rate of all available DMARDs.

Other studies, however, showed less pronounced effects of MTX. Studies reported ongoing active RA and a significant discontinuation rate due to toxicity, although the retention rate for MTX was still 50% after 5 years. However, the studies also indicated that sufficient dosing is crucial for the effectivity of MTX, as 7.5 mg MTX per week resulted in less pronounced effects and increased relapses.

Several long-term studies on mostly advanced, highly destructive, and previously largely treatment-resistant RA, showed satisfactory to good effectivity that could be maintained for years. Treatment could be continued for longer than was known for other basic therapeutic agents. In many cases, however, the disease remained active and remissions did not occur or occurred rarely.

3.1.2. Influence on life expectancy and the Ratingen long-term study

Since the middle of the last century, several studies have shown that people with RA have an increased mortality rate. The standardized mortality rate (SMR) was between 2.26 and 2.7, although the individual studies cannot be compared due to the different structure of the general population, the

Author	Year	n	Type of study	Disease duration (years)	Treatment duration in months (range)	Dose (mg per week)	Effectiveness	Per cent	After years
Kremer (2)	1992	29	prospective	11,7	90 (79-107)	11.7	good	62%	71/2
Weinblatt (3)	1992	26	prospective	8,9	84	10.2	good	46%	7
Sany (4)	1991	191	prospective	8,5	19 (3-58)	10.2	good	46%	5
Hanrahan (5)	1989	128	prospective	12	22 (1-60)	12.8	moderate	50%	5
Alarcon (6)	1989	152	prospective	9,1			good		
Mielants (7)	1991	92	prospective	11	~16	7.5	moderate		
Rau (8)	1988	271	prospective	8,5	31.4 (1-108)	12.1	good	60%	5
Krause (9)	1995	271	prospective	8,5	120 (12-198)		good		
Bologna (10)	1997	453	retrospective		35 (3-106)		good	73%	5
Weinblatt (1)	1994	123	prospective	6,5	~45		good	64%	5

Table 3.1: Long-term observational studies and reviews. **Comment**: MTX was often the last therapeutic option available for those treated, i.e. after discontinuation there was no other therapy available.

duration of the disease and the duration of observation. However, all studies show that the activity and severity of the disease, the radiological progression, the functional disability and the inability to work not only predict a poor prognosis but also a shortened life expectancy (9, 11-15).

Ratingen long-term study

The Ratingen long-term study has prospectively documented all patients who started MTX therapy at the Ratingen Rheumatology Clinic using standardized questionnaires over an average of 10 years since 1980. In addition to the effectivity of long-term therapy with MTX, this study also answered questions about the survival of those treated. At least 30% of those treated achieved remission and after 5 years 60% of those affected were still being treated with MTX. The examination at the end of the study period was documented for at least 94.5% of those treated (256 of 271) and it was shown that mortality correlated with a response to MTX after one year. After one year, 105 (39%) participants had an improvement in activity parameters of >50%, 74 participants (27%) had an improvement of 20-50%, 55 participants (20%) were unchanged and 37 participants (14%) had discontinued therapy. There was a clear relationship between the response to MTX treatment and the SMR: in the group with >50% improvement, the SMR was 1.47, in the group with 20-50% improvement it was 1.85, compared to 4.11 in the group without improvement and 5.56 in the group of patients who had discontinued treatment during the first year (9) (☞ Figure 3.1).

In 2003, a further follow-up study of the treated patients was carried out, which again showed that the best outcome was achieved by those patients who had responded best to MTX therapy after just one year (>50% improvement).

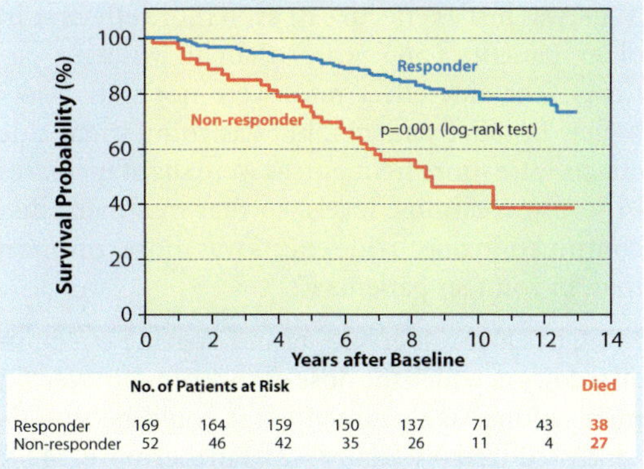

Figure 3.1: Kaplan-Meier curve of the estimated probability of survival. The groups of treated patients with improvement of >50% or 20-50% after one year are classified as responders, those treated without improvement as non-responders. The overall survival rate after 8 years was 84% for the responders and 56% for the non-responders after one year of MTX treatment (9).

Other studies have also found a positive effect of MTX therapy on survival. For example, one study showed that the unadjusted mortality rate of those treated with MTX was 0.8 compared to the group not treated with MTX. In particular, the risk of cardiovascular death was reduced to 0.3 using MTX therapy, while the risk of non-cardiovascular death was 0.6. Folic acid substitution had no effect on the risk of death. In this study, the other DMARDs used had no effect on the mortality rate (15).

The increased mortality in RA depending on disease activity – in particular cardiovascular mortality – is reduced in the long term by MTX, which correlates with the clinical effectivity of MTX.

3.2. Effectivity in old age, steroid-sparing effect

Although the term 'remission' was used much more cautiously in Rheumatology before the biologics era, and remission according to the Pinals criteria was considered almost impossible to achieve with conventional basic therapy ("RA is an incurable disease"), a considerable number of remissions were reported with MTX. Various studies report remission rates of 15 to over 60%, with the majority of studies reporting remission rates of 20 to 30% using MTX (7, 16-20).

MTX was just as effective or even more effective in older patients (>65 years) than in younger patients. The side effect rates were not statistically higher in older patients, but gastrointestinal side effects were more frequent, as were slight increases in serum creatinine levels, so that treatment discontinuation due to side effects was more common than in younger patients (21).

MTX has a considerable steroid-sparing effect: in all studies in which the dose of concomitant steroid medication was documented, it could be significantly reduced (☞ Figure 3.2). Furthermore, MTX is considered preventive with regard to the development of diabetes mellitus in patients with RA (22, 23).

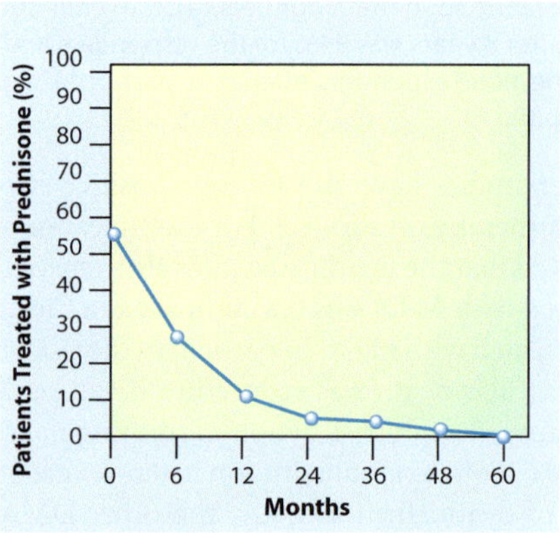

Figure 3.2: Percentage of those treated with corticosteroids in the Ratingen long-term study.

> Older and more recent studies, mostly investigating advanced cases of RA, showed surprisingly high (differently defined) remission rates of around 20-30% with MTX monotherapy. The effectivity of MTX does not decrease with age. However, an age-related reduction in creatinine clearance and thus also in MTX elimination can lead to an increase in toxicity.
>
> MTX has a pronounced steroid-sparing effect and also has a preventive effect on the development of cardiovascular events and diabetes mellitus.

3.3. Influence on functional capacity

Impairment of the patient's functional capacity at the onset of disease is mainly determined by disease activity, i.e. swelling and pain at rest and, in addition, during exertion. In later stages, restrictions due to joint destruction and deformities ensue. Since MTX reduces both the disease activity and, optimally, prevents or delays the development of destruction, it naturally also influences the functional capacity, measured with the Hannover Functional Questionnaire (FFbH) or the Health Assessment Questionnaire (HAQ). Such data were rarely considered in the past, but are now collected in nearly all studies. For example, an increase in the mean FFbH from 68 to 81 (normal function = 100) was observed using MTX. The improvement in function under MTX monotherapy was also demonstrated in comparative studies with biologics: in the TEMPO trial, after one year the HAQ (0-3) improved from 1.8 to 0.8 under the combination treatment etanercept (ETA)/MTX, from 1.7 to 1.0 in the ETA group and from 1.7 to 1.1 in the MTX group, which was also confirmed after 2 years (24). In the PREMIER study, which compared adalimumab (ADA) with MTX and the combination of both, the HAQ Disability Index improved by 1.1 in the combination group, compared to 0.8 in both the ADA and MTX monotherapy groups. After 2 years, the improvement was 1.0 in the combination group and 0.9 under ADA and MTX. After 2 years, 33% of patients in the combination group, compared with 19% in the monotherapy arms, had an HAQ DI of 0, i.e. no disability at all (25).

3.4. Duration of treatment as an indicator of effectivity

In addition to the effectivity and tolerability of MTX, long-term tolerability plays a major role in chronic diseases. The length of time during which the patient can be treated continuously with the same basic therapeutic agent can be considered a measure of its tolerability and effectivity . For "life table" analyses of the duration of use of basic therapeutic agents, data are often used from rheumatology clinics and later also from registry data. It was shown that MTX had a significantly longer "drug survival rate" compared to the other available DMARDs. While a treatment duration of 2 years or less was stated for antimalarial drugs, auranofin, intramuscular gold and D-penicillamine, the duration for MTX was 4.25 years ($p<0.005$). Similarly, the percentage of patients receiving continuously other DMARDs was 41-51% after 2 years and only 20-25% after 5 years. In contrast, these figures were 57% for MTX and 72% and 57% respectively ($p<0.01$) (26). Another long-term study showed that even after 7.5 years, 62% of participants were still receiving MTX treatment (27).

However, there were also studies that observed treatment continuation with MTX in only 25% of participants after 60 months, for which the cause could be a delayed effect. In a study on the HAQ, after initial improvement, the value returned to baseline after 8 years. The authors considered the MTX treatment to be suboptimal and called for a faster dose escalation and longer maintenance of an optimal or the highest tolerated dose (28). In a Dutch cohort of 1,022 participants, it was then shown that there was a significant relationship between the duration of treatment with MTX and folic acid substitution, the treating physician and the simultaneous administration of prednisolone. The most common reason for discontinuation was toxicity (16.7%) followed by ineffectivity (6.7%) (29).

The particularly long "drug survival time" of MTX indicates good acceptance among patients due to low toxicity and good efficacy. In addition, the dosage can be individually adjusted, whereby a dose that is too low and therefore not fully effective should be avoided.

3.5. Comparison with leflunomide

Several studies have compared leflunomide (LEF) with MTX, with varying results regarding effectivity. In a 1-year study on patients with long-standing RA, the ACR20 response and radiological progression with LEF 20 mg per day were comparable to MTX (up to 15 mg per week). Both substances were superior to the placebo arm in this placebo-controlled study (30). In another study, no ACR response was reported, but with regard to the primary endpoints of swollen and painful joints and participant and physician assessment, MTX was significantly better than LEF in the first year. However, this effect was lost in the second year and both therapies were equally effective. Nevertheless, radiological progression appeared to be somewhat lower with MTX, which must be related to a slightly higher rate of side effects with MTX (increased liver enzymes). Of note, in this study, folic acid was not regularly administered to those treated with MTX (31). Finally, a randomized study was published that compared MTX with LEF over a period of 1 year. It showed a better response to MTX in relation to all primary endpoints (swollen and painful joints, patient and physician assessment), while the difference for the secondary endpoints (morning stiffness, pain intensity, HAQ) was not statistically significant (32).

In the large studies with a total of 1800 patients, MTX appears to be somewhat more effective than LEF, especially in the first year, although the side effect rate of MTX must be taken into account.

3.6. Methotrexate monotherapy vs triple therapy

In a single-blind, randomized study, two aspects were investigated: how triple therapy (TT) compares to MTX monotherapy (MM) and which "bridging" strategy for GC therapy (single intramuscular administration or oral administration over 10 days) performs better (33). The primary endpoints were the AUC (area under the curve) for the DAS28 and the HAQ, as well as the proportion of treated patients with radiological progression. In the study design, almost 100 treated patients were randomized into 3 arms: TT with intramuscular GC, TT with oral GC, and MTX mono (MM) with oral GC. A "treat to target" strategy was pursued during the one-year phase, with a DAS28 of <2.4 being the target. If this goal was not achieved, the treatment was intensified and biologics could be included. There was no difference between the three groups in terms of radiological progression, but the AUC for the DAS28 and the HAQ was lower in the TT group than in the MM group. This meant that less intensification of antirheumatic therapy was necessary under TT. However, treatment adjustments due to side effects were also more frequent using TT than using MM. The authors conclude that the treatment goals can be achieved more quickly using TT, but radiological progression remains unchanged. With regard to GC therapy, no difference could be found between the single intramuscular administration and short-term oral therapy.

3.7. Comparison with biologics

Since MTX became established as the DMARD of choice in the treatment of RA, great progress has been made in the recent 10-15 years in understanding the pathophysiology of RA. This better understanding has led to the development of new drugs that target factors which play a defined role in the inflammatory process leading to joint destruction. Currently, the most promising principle is the inhibition of proinflammatory cytokines such as tumor necrosis factor-alpha (TNF-α), interleukin-1 (IL-1) and interleukin-6 (IL-6), the elimination of a specific population of B lymphocytes using rituximab and the modulation of cell–cell contacts of immune cells using abatacept. All of these have proven to be very effective in the treatment of RA, with their advantages being the rapid onset of action, good tolerability and the disproportionately strong inhibition of radiological progression. Because of these qualities, the new drugs were considered a "breakthrough" in the treatment of RA. As far as possible, the efficacy of these biologics as monotherapy will be compared with MTX.

3.7.1. Etanercept

The first direct comparison between etanercept (ETA) and MTX was made in the ERA (Early Rheumatoid Arthritis) study (34). 632 participants with early RA (disease duration ≤3 years) who were rheumatoid factor positive or had at least 3 erosions were randomized in a double-blind manner to receive 10 mg or 25 mg ETA twice weekly or 7.5 mg MTX per week, with the MTX dose being gradually increased to 20 mg weekly; participants also received 1 mg folic acid daily. The number of participants with an ACR20/50/70 improvement was significantly higher with ETA than with MTX during the first 6 months, with a significantly faster response, but the improvement in response rates ran parallel in the second half of the year. After 12 months, 72% of patients receiving ETA achieved an ACR20 response compared to 65% in the MTX group (p=0.16). Those included were then treated further in an open study, and even after 2 years, no significant differences were found between ETA and MTX with regard to the ACR 20/50/70 response. Even so, there was a trend towards better "drug survival" for ETA (74% for ETA vs 59% for MTX after 2 years) (35).

The very good effectivity of MTX compared to ETA has surprised experts. The slower onset of action of MTX is partially explained by the initially insufficient dose of MTX at 7.5 mg per week for a period of 4 weeks. In addition, the effectivity may have been impaired by concomitant folic acid supplementation.

Further comparisons between MTX and TNF-α inhibitors arise from the three-armed studies that compared the combination of MTX/TNF-α inhibitor with the two individual substances as monotherapy. The TEMPO study (36) was used to compare the combination of ETA+MTX with the two individual substances in 686 patients with an average duration of illness of 6.8 years who had responded unsatisfactorily to at least one basic therapeutic agent. The limitation of the study is that 42% of those included had previously received MTX and had stopped taking it for various reasons. In this study, ETA was dosed at 2 × 25 mg per week, MTX alone and in combination was started at 7.5 mg per week and only increased to 20 mg if the effect was insufficient. After one year, both the ACR20/50/70 response rates and the DAS28 improvement were lower with MTX than with ETA, but the differences were not significant, while the combination showed significantly better results than the individual substances (☞ Figure 3.3). Here, too, an extension phase of treatment was carried out, and during the second year the ACR20/50/70 response rate remained largely unchanged compared to the first year in all three treatment arms. In the monotherapy groups, with otherwise identical results, the improvement in the number of swollen and tender joints was significantly greater with ETA than with MTX. A low disease activity status (DAS <2.4) was achieved with approximately equal frequency under MTX and ETA (38.6/44.4%), and remission (DAS <1.6) was achieved more frequently using ETA (23.3%) than using MTX (15.8%) (p<0.05) (24).

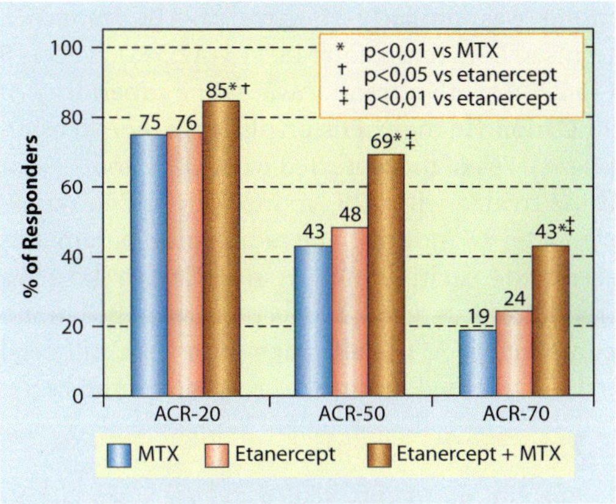

Figure 3.3: ACR20/50/70 response rates after 52 weeks in the TEMPO study (36).

3.7.2. Adalimumab

The PREMIER study (25) compared the combination of adalimumab (ADA) + MTX with the two individual components in 799 patients with an average disease duration of 0.6-0.7 years since diagnosis and high inflammatory activity. A positive rheumatoid factor or at least one erosion was also required as an inclusion criterion. In the case of insufficient response, MTX (with folic acid supplementation) could be increased from 7.5 mg per week to 15 mg by week 8 and to 20 mg in week 9. The ADA dose could also be increased to weekly doses in patients who did not achieve an ACR20, but this only had a minor impact on efficacy.

After one year, 41% achieved an ACR50 response with ADA and 46% with MTX, which was not statistically significant. Comparing monotherapies, there were no statistically significant clinical and compliance-related advantages for MTX over ADA. After 2 years, the response rates achieved in the first year were essentially maintained (☞ Figure 3.4).

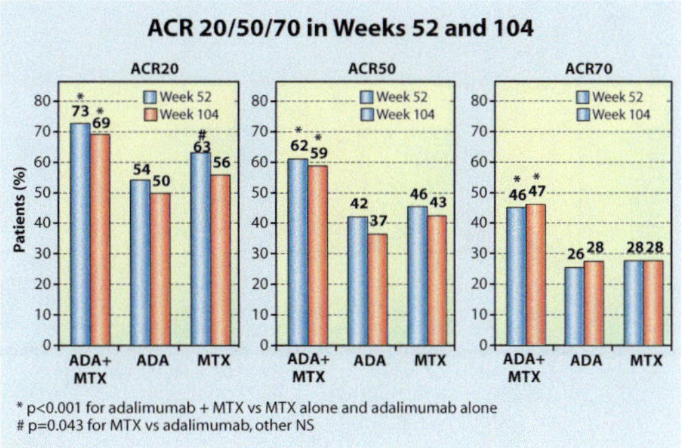

Figure 3.4: ACR20/50/70 response rates in the PREMIER study over 52 weeks (25).

A relatively high number of participants achieved remission, defined as DAS28 <2.6 with 23% of the ADA monotherapy group and 21% of the MTX monotherapy group (p<0.001). After two years, the number of remissions had even increased slightly among the completers.

The PREMIER study was further evaluated from various perspectives. The influence on radiological progression was also of interest, as reported in another publication (37). It was shown that with increasing inflammatory activity over time, there was an increase in erosions and joint space narrowing. This occurred predominantly in the monotherapy groups, although the authors also divided the participants into tertials of DAS28 activity. There were no differences between ADA and MTX in terms of the absolute number and percentage of patients treated in the DAS28 tertials. However, in the groups with low DAS28 activity in particular, there was significantly less radiological progression with ADA monotherapy compared with the MTX group (☞ Figure 3.5).

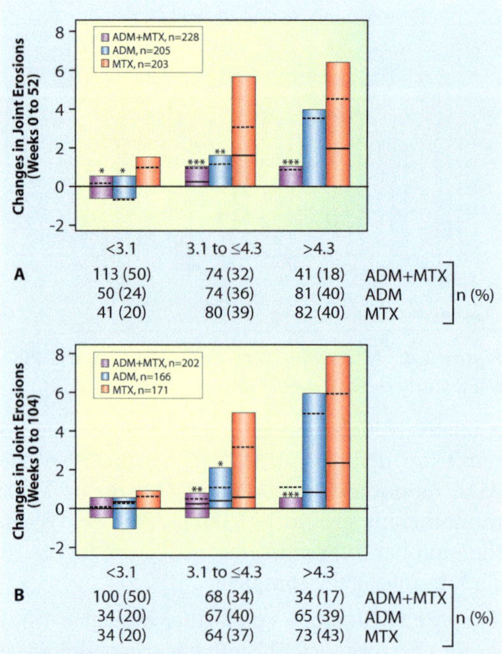

Figure 3.5: Changes in joint erosions (JE) related to inflammatory activity over time (DAS28-CRP; TA-DAS28 (CRP) = time averaged DAS28-CRP). Participants were divided into tertials, the figure shows the results after 52 weeks (**A**) and 104 weeks (**B**).
*p<0.05 significance level for the difference between the treatment group and MTX monotherapy;
**p<0.01; ***p<0.001. The figure shows the median (solid line), mean (dashed line) and the interquartile range (bars). ADA = Adalimumab (37).

3.7.3. Abatacept

In a randomized, double-blind IIIb study, abatacept (ABC) SC as monotherapy was compared with ABC in combination with MTX and MTX monotherapy (38). The study ran for 1 year, after which participants with low disease activity (DAS28-CRP <3.2) were transferred to an extension phase in which all RA medications were discontinued. The primary endpoints were DAS28-CRP <2.6 after 1 year and after 1 year and 18 months. This study was conducted on patients with early RA (disease duration <2 years) who had DAS28-CRP ≥3.2 and were positive for ACPA-2 antibodies. Almost 120 patients were included in each group and although the primary endpoint was the comparison of ABC+MTX versus MTX mono, comparisons could also be made between the monotherapy arms. After one year, MTX mono was similarly effective as ABC mono in terms of DAS remission (48/113 (42.5%) vs 52/115 (45.2%)), with a trend towards the superiority of ABC mono in the extension phase. In the extension phase, 17% of those treated with MTX and 28% of those treated with ABC mono were still in remission after 18 months. The radiological parameters recorded (osteitis, synovitis in MRI) also showed a trend towards greater effectivity of ABC mono compared to MTX, although these data still need to be confirmed in further prospective studies.

3.7.4. Tocilizumab

In one study, tocilizumab 8 mg/kg body weight (TCZ) every 4 weeks intravenously was compared with MTX in RA patients who had not yet failed treatment with MTX or a biologic. This was a 24-week study in which a double-blind, double-dummy, parallel group design was chosen (39). In this study, MTX was titrated from 7.5 mg per week to 20 mg per week within 8 weeks and a third arm was also included in which the participants received placebo for the first 8 weeks and were then switched to TCZ 8 mg/kg body weight every four weeks. A total of 673 patients were included, of which 101 participants were in the group that initially received placebo. The primary endpoint was an ACR20 response after 24 weeks. Here, TCZ performed significantly better, with an ACR20 response in 69.9% of participants versus 52.5% under MTX. Further analyses also showed a statistically better ACR50 and ACR70 response for TCZ compared to MTX (ACR50: 44.1% versus 33.5%; ACR70: 28.0% versus 15.1%). Regarding the side effects observed, more participants under TCZ had grade 3 neutropenia and increased lipid levels, while increases in liver transaminases over three times the norm occurred less frequently under TCZ.

In the FUNCTION study, patients with TCZ monotherapy were compared with MTX+placebo. The dose of MTX was increased according to the above-mentioned study. Significantly better functionality and less radiographic progression in the vdH score were observed over 2 years. An increased number of serious infections was considered an additional risk (40). A side effect that appears to occur significantly more frequently with TCZ than with MTX is colon perforation (41).

MTX monotherapy (with folic acid supplementation) is almost comparable to monotherapy with ETA and adalimumab in terms of its clinical effectivity, with ETA being numerically slightly better and ADA slightly worse than MTX, but in each case not statistically significant. Direct comparisons of MTX with infliximab are currently lacking. TCZ proved to be significantly more effective than MTX, albeit at the cost of a slightly higher rate of side effects. In ABC, too, monotherapy appears to be slightly more effective than MTX, although these data still need to be confirmed in a prospective study.

3.8. New substances, small molecules

MTX has achieved a very high status as an initial treatment in RA and it serves as a reference drug in the investigation of new drugs for the treatment of RA. In recent years, new drugs have been approved, all of which belong to the class of JAK inhibitors.

3.8.1. Tofacitinib

In a 24-month study, tofacitinib (TFB) was investigated in two doses (2 × 5 mg/day or 2 × 10 mg per day) and compared with MTX in patients with RA who had not yet received MTX (randomization 2:2:1). MTX was increased to 20 mg per week within 8 weeks. The primary endpoints reported here were changes in the modified vdH-Sharp score and the proportion of participants with an ACR70 response (42). 956 participants were randomized and evaluated, and the first results were compared after 6 months. TFB was shown to have a greater impact on radiological progression than MTX (mean dose 18.5 mg per week), but changes in the vdH Sharp score were small and did not reach a minimal difference of clinical significance (equivalent to 4.6 points = 1% of the modified vdH Sharp score). Clinical response was better for both TFB doses than for MTX, as significantly more ACR70 responses were achieved in the TFB group than in the MTX group (TFB 5 mg 25.5 ± 2.3%, TFB 10 mg 37.7 ± 2.4%, MTX 12.0 ± 2.4%; $p<0.001$ for each TFB group). Regarding physical function, a significantly better performance was also found for both TFB doses for both the HAQ-DI and FACIT scores. However, certain side effects also occurred more frequently with TFB, such as neutropenia, lymphopenia, an increase in LDL cholesterol or creatinine, leading the authors to conclude that the better efficacy of TFB must be weighed up with the slightly higher rate of side effects.

3.8.2. Baricitinib

Fleischmann et al. compared the efficacy of baricitinib (BAR) versus MTX monotherapy in a phase III study on 588 csDMARD-naive RA patients. At week 24, baricitinib showed a significantly higher ACR20 response (77%) than MTX (62%) and a significant difference in terms of SDAI remission. There was also a significant improvement in function, measured using the HAQ-DI. With regard to radiological progression, BAR monotherapy was not significantly better in the modified vdH/Sharp score than MTX monotherapy. Another advantage was seen in the rapid response from week 1, which was rated as significantly better over the course up to week 52 than with MTX monotherapy (43).

3.8.3. Upadacitinib

Upadacitinib (UPA) was compared with MTX monotherapy in 947 MTX-naive patients with early RA as part of the SELECT-EARLY study. In all respects, UPA monotherapy was shown to be superior in both doses compared to MTX monotherapy. UPA led to significantly better results in the ACR20 (after 12 weeks: UPA 30 mg 77%, UPA 15 mg 76%, MTX 20 mg 54%, after 24 weeks: UPA 30 mg 78%, UPA 15 mg 79%, MTX 20 mg 59%) as early as week 2, although it should be noted that the MTX dose was initially increased over 8 weeks (from 7.5/10 mg to 17.5/20 mg). From week 2 onwards, the HAQ-DI values were significantly better with UPA monotherapy than in the MTX group. The proportion of prevented radiographic progression in the sense of a modified Sharp score = 0 was significantly higher with UPA monotherapy than with MTX monotherapy (UPA 15 mg 88%, UPA 30 mg 89% versus 78% in the MTX arm). However, infections and herpes zoster were observed significantly more frequently in the UPA arms than with MTX monotherapy (44).

Recently, the results of the long term extension study of the SELECT-EARLY study were published (van Vollenhoven R, Strand V, Takeuchi T et al. Upadacitinib monotherapy versus methotrexate monotherapy in patients with rheumatoid arthritis: efficacy and safety through 5 years in the SELECT-EARLY randomized controlled trial. Arthritis Research & Therapy 2024;26:143-158). After 5 years it could be shown that higher proportions of patients consistently achieved disease activity targets with upadacitinib than MTX. With upadacitinib 15/30 mg 53%/59% of patients attained CDAI remission versus 43% with MTX at week 260. Further analyses showed better CDAI, DAS28(CRP), and ACR responses with upadacitinib relative to MTX at week 260. Upadacitinib treatment also resulted in numerically greater inhibition of structural joint progression through week 260 compared to MTX. Rates of serious infections, herpes zoster, creatine phosphokinase elevation, nonmelanoma skin cancer, and neutropenia were numerically higher with upadacitinib than MTX. The observed safety profile of upadacitinib over 5 years was consistent with earlier trial results and integrated phase 3 safety analyses.

3.8.4. Filgotinib

The FINCH 3 study investigated the efficacy of filgotinib (FIL) + MTX in two different doses and FIL monotherapy versus MTX monotherapy. Here, FIL resulted in a significantly better response than MTX in the ACR50/70, the SDAI and the CDAI as early as week 24; however, there were no significant differences in ACR20. A significantly better result was reported with FIL monotherapy (200 mg) in terms of radiographic progression (determined by the mTSS; FIL monotherapy 0.23 versus 0.74 MTX monotherapy) (45).

3.8.5. Side effects of JAK inhibitors

It is suspected that there is a higher rate of herpes zoster infections, particularly in Japanese and South Korean patients, as well as an increased rate of venous thromboembolic events (46). Since the issuing of the dear doctor letter for all JAK inhibitors in 2023 following the ORAL Surveillance study (47), there is still an ongoing discussion about the true safety aspects of this drug class when used in chronic inflammatory diseases.This is reflected by continuous updates, especially for Europe, which result in more realistic rather than the very restrictive statements formulated in the 2023 dear doctor letter (www.dgrh.de/Januskinase-Inhibitoren (JAKi) 2024, 48,49).

> "Small molecules", of which JAK inhibitors in particular are considered promising, have been increasingly approved as monotherapy for RA in recent years. In the large-scale studies, a significant improvement in remission and, in particular, in terms of radiological progression was found for the drugs mentioned, BAR, UPA and FIL. However, since there is also a significantly increased risk of herpes zoster infections and an increased risk of thromboembolism, the indication must be determined on an individual basis.

3.9. References

1. Weinblatt ME, Kaplan H, Germain BF, et al. Methotrexate in rheumatoid arthritis: a five year prospective multicenter trial. Arthritis Rheum 1994;37:1492-8

2. Kremer JM, Phelps CT. Long-term prospective study of the use of methotrexate in the treatment of rheumatoid arthritis. Arthritis Rheum 1992;35:138-145

3. Weinblatt ME, Weissman BN, Holdsworth DE, Fraser PA, Maier AL, et al. Long-term prospective study of methotrexate in the treatment of rheumatoid arthritis. 84-month update. Arthritis Rheum 1992;35:129-37

4. Sany J, Anaya JM, Lussiez V, Couret M, Combe B et al. Treatment of rheumatoid arthritis with methotrexate: a prospective open long term study of 191 cases. J Rheumatol 1991;18:1323-7

5. Hanrahan PS, Scrivens GA, Russell AS. Prospective long term follow-up of methotrexate therapy in rheumatoid arthritis: Toxicity, efficacy and radiological progression. Brit J Rheum 1989;28:147-53

6. Alarcon GS, Tracy IC, Blackburn WD Jr. Methotrexate in rheumatoid arthritis: toxic effects as the major factor in limiting long-term treatment. Arthritis Rheum 1989; 32:671-6

7. Mielants H, Veys EM, van der Straeten C, Ackerman C, Goemaere S. The efficacy and toxicity of a constant low dose of methotrexate as a treatment for intractable rheumatoid arthritis: An open prospective study. J Rheumatol 1991;18:978-83

8. Rau R, Schleusser B, Herborn G, Karger T. Long-term treatment of destructive rheumatoid arthritis with methotrexate. J Rheumatol 1997;24:1881-89

9. Krause D, Schleusser B, Herborn G, Rau R. Response to methotrexate treatment is associated with reduced mortality in patients with severe rheumatoid arthritis. Arthritis Rheum 2000;43:14-21

10. Bologna C, Viu P, Picot MC et al. Long-term follow-up of 453 rheumatoid arthritis patients treated with methotrexate: an open, retrospective, observational study. Br J Rheumatol 1997;36:535-540

11. Cobb S, Anderson F, Bauer W. Length of life and cause of death in rheumatoid arthritis. N Engl J Med 1953;249:553-6

12. Mutru O, Laakso M, Isomäki HA, Koota K. Ten year mortality and causes of death in patients with rheumatoid arthritis. BMJ 1985;290:1797-9

13. Wolfe F, Mitchell DM, Sibley JT, Fries JF, Bloch DA, Williams CA, et al. The mortality of rheumatoid arthritis. Arthritis Rheum 1994;37:481-94

14. Simmons DPM, Jones MA, Scott DL, Prior P. Longterm mortality outcome in patients with rheumatoid arthritis: early presenters continue to do well. JRheumatol 1998;25:1072-7

15. Choi HK, Hernan MA, Seeger JD, et al. Methotrexate and mortality in patients with rheumatoid arthritis: a prospective study. Lancet 2002;359:1173-7

16. Karger T, Rau R. Methotrexat-Behandlung hochaktiver chronischer Polyarthritiden. Münch Med Wschr 1984; 126:560

17. Rau R, Herborn G, Karger T, Werdier D. Retardation of radiologic progression in rheumatoid arthritis with methotrexate therapy. Arthritis Rheum 1991;10:1236-44

18. Drosos AA, Karantanas AH, Psychos D, Tsampoulas C, Moutsopulos HM: Can treatment with methotrexate influence the radiological progression of rheumatoid arthritis? Clin Rheumatol 1990;9:342-5

19. Weinstein A, Marlowe S, Korn J, Farouhar F. Effect of methotrexate on rheumatoid arthritis: A systematic analysis of 21 patients. Rheumatology 1986;9:148

20. Rau R, Karger T. Klinische Erfahrungen und Differentialindikationen der Therapie mit Methotrexat bei chronischer Polyarthritis. Internistische Welt 1987;12: 335-348

21. Köller MD, Aletaha D, Funovits J, Pangan A, Baker D, Smolen JS. Response of elderly patients with rheumatoid arthritis to methotrexate or TNF inhibitors compared with younger patients. Rheumatology 2009;48:1575-1580

22. Sun KJ, Liu LL, Hu JH, Chen YY, Xu DY. Methotrexate can prevent cardiovascular events in patients with rheumatoid arthritis: An updated meta-analysis. Medicine (Baltimore). 2021;100(7):e24579

23. Baghdadi LR. Effect of methotrexate use on the development of type 2 diabetes in rheumatoid arthritis patients: A systematic review and meta-analysis. PLoS One 2020;15(7): e0235637

24. van der Heijde D, Klareskog L, Rodriguez-Valverde V, Codreanu C et al. Comparison of etanercept and methotrexate, alone and combined, in the treatment of rheumatoid arthritis: two-year clinical and radiographic results from the TEMPO Study. A double-blind, randomised trial. Arthritis Rheum 2006;54:1063-1074

25. Breedveld F, Weisman M, Kavanaugh A, Cohen B, et al. The PREMIER Study. A multicenter, randomized, double-blind clinical trial of combination therapy with adalimumab plus methotrexate versus methotrexate alone or adalimumab alone in patients with early, aggressive rheumatoid arthritis who had not had previous methotrexate treatment. Arthritis Rheum 2006;54:26-37

26. Pincus T, Callahan LF. Methotrexate is significantly more likely to be continued over two years than gold salts, penicillamine or hydroxychloroquine in rheumatoid arthritis. Arthritis Rheum 1989;32:128

27. Morand EF, McCloud PI, Littlejohn GO. Life table analysis of 879 treatment episodes with slow acting antirheumatic drugs in community rheumatology practice. J Rheumatol 1992;19:704-8

28. Ortendahl M, Holmes T, Schettler JD, Fries JF. The methotrexate therapeutic response in rheumatoid arthritis. J Rheumatol 2002;29:2084-91

29. Hoekstra M, van de Laar MAFJ, Bernelot Moens HJ, Kruijsen MWM, Haagsma CJ. Long term observational study of methotrexate use in a Dutch cohort of 1022 patients with rheumatoid arthritis. J Rheumatol 2003; 30:2325-9

30. Strand V, Cohen S, Schiff M, Weaver A, Fleischmann R, Cannon G, Fox R, Moreland L, Olsen N, Furst D, Caldwell J, Kaine J, Sharp J, Hurley F, Loew-Friedrich I. Treatment of active rheumatoid arthritis with leflunomide compared with placebo and methotrexate. Leflunomide Rheumatoid Arthritis Investigators Group. Arch Intern Med 1999; 159: 2542-50

31. Emery P, Breedveld FC, Lemmel EM, Kaltwasser JP, Dawes PT, Gömör B, Van Den Bosch F, Nordström D, Bjorneboe O, Dahl R, Horslev-Petersen K, Rodriguez DeLa Serna A, Molloy M, Tikly M, Oed C, Rosenburg R, Loew-Friedrich I. A comparison of the efficacy and safety of leflunomide and methotrexate for the treatment of rheumatoid arthritis. Rheumatology 2000;39:655-65

32. Ishaq M, Muhammad JS, Hameed K, Mirza AI. Leflunomide or methotrexate? Comparison of clinical efficacy and safety in low socio-economic rheumatoid arthritis patients. Mod Rheumatol 2011;21:375-80

33. de Jong PH, Hazes JM, Han HK, Huisman M, van Zeben D, van der Lubbe PA, Gerards AH, van Schaeybroeck B, de Sonnaville PB, van Krugten MV, Luime JJ, Weel AE. Randomised comparison of initial triple DMARD therapy with methotrexate monotherapy in combination with low-dose glucocorticoid bridging therapy; 1-year data of the tREACH trial. Ann Rheum Dis 2014; 73:1331-9

34. Bathon JM, Martin RW, Fleischmann RM, Tesser JR, Schiff MH, Keystone ES, Genovese MC, Wasko MC, Moreland LW, Weaver AL, Markenson J, Finck BK. A comparison of etanercept and methotrexate in patients with early rheumatoid arthritis. N Engl J Med 2000; 343:1586-93

35. Genovese M, Bathon J, Martin R, Fleischmann R, et al. Etanercept versus methotrexate in patients with early rheumatoid arthritis. Two-year radiographic and clinical outcomes. Arthritis Rheum 2002;45:1443-50

36. Klareskog L, van der Heijde D, de Jager JP, Gough A, Kalden J, Malaise M, Martin Mola E, Pavelka K, Sany J, Settas L, Wajdula J, Pedersen R, Fatenejad S, Sanda M; TEMPO (Trial of Etanercept and Methotrexate with Radiographic Patient Outcomes) study investigators. Therapeutic effect of the combination of etanercept and methotrexate compared with each treatment alone in patients with rheumatoid arthritis: double-blind randomised controlled trial. Lancet 2004;363:675-81

37. Smolen JS, van der Heijde DM, Keystone EC, van Vollenhoven RF, Goldring MB, Guérette B, Cifaldi MA, Chen N, Liu S, Landewé RB. Association of joint space narrowing with impairment of physical function and work ability in patients with early rheumatoid arthritis: protection beyond disease control by adalimumab plus methotrexate. Ann Rheum Dis 2013;72:1156-62

38. Emery P, Burmester GR, Bykerk VP, Combe BG, Furst DE, Barré E, Karyekar CS, Wong DA, Huizinga TW. Evaluating drug-free remission with abatacept in early rheumatoid arthritis: results from the phase 3b, multicentre, randomised, active-controlled AVERT study of 24 months, with a 12-

month, double-blind treatment period. Ann Rheum Dis 2015;74:19-26

39. Jones G, Sebba A, Gu J, Lowenstein MB, Calvo A, Gomez-Reino JJ, Siri DA, Tomsic M, Alecock E, Woodworth T, Genovese MC. Comparison of tocilizumab monotherapy versus methotrexate monotherapy in patients with moderate to severe rheumatoid arthritis: the AMBITION study. Ann Rheum Dis 2010;69:88-96

40. Burmester GR, Rigby WF, van Vollenhoven RF, Kay J, Rubbert-Roth A, Blanco R, Kadva A, Dimonaco S. Tocilizumab combination therapy or monotherapy or methotrexate monotherapy in methotrexate-naive patients with early rheumatoid arthritis: 2-year clinical and radiographic results from the randomised, placebo-controlled FUNCTION trial. Ann Rheum Dis. 2017;76(7): 1279-1284

41. Strangfeld A, Richter A, Siegmund B, et al. Risk for lower intestinal perforations in patients with rheumatoid arthritis treated with tocilizumab in comparison to treatment with other biologic or conventional synthetic DMARDs; Annals of the Rheumatic Diseases 2017;76: 504-510

42. Lee EB, Fleischmann R, Hall S, Wilkinson B, Bradley JD, Gruben D, Koncz T, Krishnaswami S, Wallenstein GV, Zang C, Zwillich SH, van Vollenhoven RF; ORALStart Investigators. Tofacitinib versus methotrexate in rheumatoid arthritis. N Engl J Med 2014;370:2377-86

43. Fleischmann R, Schiff M, van der Heijde D, RamosRemus C, Spindler A, Stanislav M, Zerbini CA, Gurbuz S, Dickson C, de Bono S, Schlichting D, Beattie S, Kuo WL, Rooney T, Macias W, Takeuchi T. Baricitinib, methotrexate, or combination in patients with rheumatoid arthritis and no or limited prior disease-modifying antirheumatic drug treatment. Arthritis Rheumatol 2017; 69(3):506-517

44. van Vollenhoven R, Takeuchi T, Pangan AL, Friedman A, Mohamed MF, Chen S, Rischmueller M, Blanco R, Xavier RM, Strand V. Efficacy and safety of upadacitinib monotherapy in methotrexate-naive patients with moderately-to-severely active rheumatoid arthritis (SELECT-EARLY): A multicenter, multi-country, randomized, double-blind, active comparator-controlled trial. Arthritis Rheumatol 2020;72(10):1607-1620

45. Westhovens R, Rigby WFC, van der Heijde D et al. Filgotinib in combination with methotrexate or as monotherapy versus methotrexate monotherapy in patients with active rheumatoid arthritis and limited or no prior exposure to methotrexate: the phase 3, randomised controlled FINCH 3 trial. Annals of the Rheumatic Diseases 2021;80:727-738

46. Sepriano A, Kerschbaumer A, Smolen JS et al. Safety of synthetic and biological DMARDs: a systematic literature review informing the 2019 update of the EULAR recommendations for the management of rheumatoid arthritis. Annals of the Rheumatic Diseases 2020;79:760-770

47. Ytterberg SR, Bhatt DL, Mikuls TR, Koch GG, Fleischmann R, Rivas JL, Germino R, Menon S, Sun Y, Wang C, Shapiro AB, Kanik KS, Connell CA; ORAL Surveillance Investigators. Cardiovascular and cancer risk with tofacitinib in rheumatoid arthritis. N Engl J Med 2022;386(4):316-326.

48. Alessandro Tomelleri, Giovanni Benanti, Adriana Cariddi, Stefania Laura Calvisi, Elena Baldissera, Nicola Boffini, Marco Matucci-Cerinic, Lorenzo DagnaThe impact of 2023 EMA recommendations on patients treated with JAK inhibitors: real-life experience from a prospective monocentric cohort. Rheumatology 2024;63:e39–e42.

49. Aymon R, Mongin D, Bergstra SA, Choquette D, Codreanu C, De Cock D, Dreyer L, Elkayam O, Huschek D, Hyrich KL, Iannone F, Inanc N, Kearsley-Fleet L, Koca SS, Kvien TK, Leeb BF, Lukina G, Nordström DC, Pavelka K, Pombo-Suarez M, Rodrigues A, Rotar Z, Strangfeld A, Verschueren P, Westermann R, Zavada J, Courvoisier DS, Finckh A, Lauper K.Evaluation of discontinuation for adverse events of JAK inhibitors and bDMARDs in an international collaboration of rheumatoid arthritis registers (the 'JAK-pot' study). Ann Rheum Dis 2024;83(4):421-428.

4. Methotrexate as a component of combination therapy for rheumatoid arthritis

Combination therapy for rheumatoid arthritis (RA) often includes the use of glucocorticoids (GC), non-steroidal anti-inflammatory drugs (NSAIDs) and potentially other non-NSAID analgesics, osteoporosis drugs and varying substances in addition to the disease modifying antirheumatic drugs (DMARDs). The following chapter deals exclusively with DMARD combination therapy for RA. The studies cited and referred to represent a selection, with priority given to randomized controlled studies (where available).

> MTX is the gold standard among conventional DMARDs (csDMARDs) in both monotherapy and combination therapy.

This is reflected in the fact that only few csDMARD combination studies were carried out without MTX. Likewise, a combination of biologics (bDMARDs) with csDMARDs is occasionally used in practice with other partners such as leflunomide, but there is neither evidence of benefit from randomized studies nor a drug approval, which frequently leads to recourse from health insurances. In contrast, there is a large amount of evidence for the benefit of MTX as a combination partner stemming from trials, which are the content of this chapter. The results of a number of earlier publications which are no longer available digitally were taken from the chapter on combination therapy in the previous edition of this book (1). In general, it must be taken into account that the measures of disease activity commonly used today, such as the DAS28, were not applied or were not yet available in studies carried out before 2000. Secondly, most studies at the time treated patients with a long duration of illness and very severe disease.

It should also be noted that a large proportion of the studies were carried out with oral MTX, and, especially somewhat older studies, with low MTX dosages by today's standards. Furthermore, the significance of the results in control groups (MTX + placebo) is partly reduced by the fact that the studies were carried out on patients with an inadequate response to MTX before the start of the trial.

4.1. Studies with MTX/csDMARD combinations that are no longer or rarely used today

- + Azathioprine (AZA)
- + D-penicillamine
- + Gold
- + Ciclosporin A (CsA)

4.1.1. Azathioprine and D-penicillamine / bucillamine

McCarthy was the first author to publish large case series with csDMARD combinations in the late 1980s and early 1990s. In 1995, after an open case series with different combinations, he presented an RA cohort with 169 rheumatoid factor (RF)-positive patients who were treated openly for at least one year with combinations containing MTX and/or AZA and hydroxychloroquine (HCQ) (2). Almost all parameters measured at that time improved significantly, the mean prednisolone dose was reduced from 9.3 to 5.9 mg, and 43% of patients achieved ACR remission. In 1989, a further case analysis of 20 patients treated with the combination MTX + AZA + HCQ showed a marked improvement after an average observation period of more than one year (3).

The first MTX+AZA combination study conducted under controlled conditions compared this combination with the two monotherapies over 24 and 48 weeks (4). The significance was limited by the small number of cases (only 110 patients reached the 48th week) and an overly cautious dose reduction in the combination by today's standards (maximum 7.5 mg per week MTX and 100 mg AZA daily); in the monotherapy groups, 15 mg per week or 150 mg daily could be given. Against this background, the combination proved to be no better than the monotherapies (AZA 26%, MTX 45%), with 38% responders (at least 30% improvement in at least 3/4 parameters). After this study, no further studies were conducted to investigate this combination.

D-penicillamine and bucillamine are not or no longer used as DMARDs in Germany, so they are only mentioned for historical reasons. Experience with the combination MTX + D-penicillamine has only been published once. In a retrospective case series in 1990, 16 patients were presented who received this combination for 5-86 months; 12 cases were evaluable (5). In no case was treatment discontinued due to adverse effects; all patients showed a significant improvement in the parameters determined (including joint count, morning stiffness, ESR, GC requirement), and 66% achieved ACR remission. In addition, the combination of MTX with bucillamine, chemically related to penicillamine, which has only been studied and used in Japan, should be mentioned. The combination was shown to be superior to the two monotherapies in a randomized controlled study with only 71 patients over 96 weeks (6). The ACR20 response in the combination group was significantly higher at 79% than with MTX (44%) and bucillamine (46%). Radiological progression was also lower, but tolerability was the same.

4.1.2. Gold

Gold is no longer available orally or parenterally as a DMARD in Germany. For historical reasons, the most important studies are presented here. In a solitary randomized controlled study, the combination of MTX + auranofin was compared with the two monotherapies in 335 patients over 48 weeks (7). MTX was significantly underdosed by today's standards at 7.5 mg per week in combination and monotherapy. Against this background, the validity of the study, which showed a significant improvement in all groups without difference, is severely limited. There was a high dropout rate of 34-40%.

A combination of MTX with parenteral gold was first reported in a publication by the Ratingen working group on the long-term use of MTX (8). Under open conditions, MTX monotherapy (n=97) and the addition of MTX to ongoing, insufficiently effective gold treatment (n=126) were compared. The initial MTX dose was most often 15-25 mg per week parenterally. The clinical results did not differ significantly in the two groups (e.g. Swollen Joint Count (SJC) after 0/12/24/36 months under MTX at 16.8/8.1/7.1/5.8, under combination 19.3/9/8.5/6.6). The discontinuation rate after one year was 17% (mono) and 10% (combination), and the frequency of adverse effects did not differ significantly. The initial conclusion from the data was that this combination offers no additional benefit compared to MTX monotherapy. The annual increase in X-ray progression also did not differ in the long term, but a later analysis showed that the annual progression before initiation of therapy was twice as high in the combination group as in the monotherapy group. Presumably, the combination group included more seriously ill patients, which puts the equivalence of mono/combination therapy into perspective.

A 48-week randomized controlled study published in 2003 compared the combination MTX + intramuscular gold vs MTX + placebo in (albeit only) 65 patients with inadequate response to MTX (9). Here, the combination proved to be clearly superior, with the ACR20, 50 and 70 responses being 61/26/21%, compared to 30/4/0% for MTX mono, and the dropout rate being 9 vs 14 patients. In addition to the small number of patients, the significance of the study is reduced by the fact that all patients had previously not responded well to MTX.

4.1.3. Ciclosporin A

Ciclosporin A (CsA) is also rarely used as a DMARD in RA today. In 148 patients with inadequate response to MTX (mean dose 10.2 mg), the combination MTX + CsA was compared with MTX + placebo in a randomized controlled study over 24 weeks (10). The combination was significantly superior to continued MTX therapy (+ placebo) in all efficacy parameters examined, with the ACR20 response being 48 vs 16%, and the improvement in TJC and SJC being 25% higher in the combination group. 17 vs 12 patients ended the study early; serum creatinine increased by an average of 0.14 mg/dl in the combination group and 0.05 mg/dl in the monotherapy group. The combination group was treated openly for a further 24 weeks, the monotherapy group switched to combination (11). 87% of the patients treated in the second half of the year remained in the study until week 48. The clinical improvement was maintained when the combination was continued, and the patients with switch achieved a similar success after 48 weeks.

In a further study, 100 CsA and MTX-naive patients were randomized to CsA + MTX vs CsA + placebo over 48 weeks; the MTX dose was initially

7.5 mg per week and could be increased to 15 mg (12). The combination was superior in the ACR20/50/70 response with 57/48/20% compared to CsA monotherapy with 47/25/12%, but only significantly so in the ACR50. The slowing of radiological progression was also significantly better (increase in the Larsen score 2.0 to 4.0 vs 2.5 to 10). The discontinuation rate was the same in both groups, but discontinuation due to ineffectivity was significantly lower in the combination with 14 vs 21.

More recently, the combination of CsA + MTX was used in two more modern studies. In the CARDERA study, 467 patients were treated with MTX + placebo, MTX + prednisolone, MTX + CsA or MTX + CsA + prednisolone in a randomized controlled trial over two years (13). Compared with MTX + placebo, both MTX + CsA and MTX + prednisolone, but MTX + CsA + prednisolone proved to be more effective in slowing down destruction (primary endpoint), and functional status and quality of life parameters also improved the most in the triple combination. However, this combination also resulted in the most toxicity-related discontinuations, but not more SAEs. In the CIMESTRA study, *de novo* MTX + placebo and MTX + CsA were compared in 160 patients over an initial period of 52 weeks in a randomized controlled trial (14). The dosage could be increased to 20 mg per week for MTX and to 4 mg/kg body weight for CsA. As a special feature, betamethasone injections into swollen joints were possible and were carried out intensively. The combination was only superior in a few of the parameters recorded; overall, the study conducted on early RA led to excellent results, e.g. ACR20 response 85% (combination) or 68% (mono) with almost completely halted radiological progression. The open extension data over five years continued to show minimal progression and a DAS remission in 78% of patients (15).

The studies presented in this chapter for historical reasons no longer play a role in the German healthcare system, although the MTX combinations with parenteral gold and CsA were characterized by good efficacy (albeit in some cases the safety profile was problematic). It is not expected that these combinations will regain importance in the future, given the many treatment options available today.

4.2. Studies with commonly used MTX-csDMARD combinations

- + Leflunomide (LEF)
- + Sulfasalazine (SSZ)
- + Hydroxychloroquine (HCQ)

4.2.1. Leflunomide

The importance of csDMARD combination therapies has declined significantly over the last ten years in view of the many other effective options, as the annual evaluations of the DRFZ from the “Kerndokumentation“ data show (see also below). Among the more frequently used combinations, the combination MTX + leflunomide is the most common, whilst only tested in a few studies. The most important basis for this is a randomized controlled study in which 263 patients with a long duration of illness (average 11.6 years) and inadequate response to MTX were initially treated with MTX + LEF vs MTX + placebo for 24 weeks (16). MTX was dosed orally at 10-15 mg per week, LEF after a loading dose of 10 mg daily and optionally increased to 20 mg. The combination was shown to be significantly superior (examples: ACR20 response 46 vs 20%, ACR70 response 10 vs 2%). This also applied to the HAQ and the SF36. Discontinuation rates and frequency of AEs did not differ in the two groups. However, increases in TA were more common in the combination group (therefore discontinuation in three vs one patient). In an open 24-week extension (17), the combination patients maintained this response with a slight further increase in the rate, the MTX patients switched to MTX + LEF and finally achieved a similar response (ACR20 response week 48: 59 vs 57%). Increases in liver enzymes were less common in the second half of the year and no longer led to discontinuation. More recently, the combination was investigated in an open study with 74 patients in a more cautious dosage with LEF 10 mg per day without loading dose, MTX orally with a starting dose of 7.5 mg per week with optional increase to 15 mg (18). 65/74 patients reached the end of the study after 20 weeks with an ACR20 response of 72%, reduction of SJC by 12 and improvement of HAQ by 0.65. Four patients had to discontinue therapy with SAE, 22% showed increases in transaminases (TA) (including two discontinuations, normalization after discontinuation). A prospective Chinese cohort study compared the combinations MTX + LEF and MTX + HCQ over two years with surprising results (19). MTX + HCQ showed a significantly higher remission rate at the endpoint (47 vs. 33%) and also better results in the other endpoints, with equally good tolerability for both combinations. However, these results should be interpreted with caution due to the open design. CARERA, a recent comparative study with various starting therapies, also included the combination MTX + LEF, which is discussed below.

The FDA recently issued a Black Box Warning in 2010 to highlight the increased hepatotoxic risk when combining LEF with other potentially liver-damaging drugs, including MTX (20). They reported 49 cases of severe liver damage during ongoing LEF therapy collected between 2002 and 2009, including 14 deaths. 46 of 49 patients had taken other hepatotoxic drugs, including MTX. Since the German product information often warns against the combination of MTX + LEF, the prescription of this widely used combination requires careful patient information.

In addition to TA increases, cytopenias and pneumonitis have occasionally been reported in individual cases in small case series with the combination MTX + LEF (as well as with monotherapies) (21). It is not yet clear whether these complications occur more frequently with the combination than with monotherapies. They generally occur more frequently in Southeast Asia than in Europe. In the retrospective Australian SMILE study, the safety of MTX-mono, LEF-mono, MTX + LEF and other DMARDs was investigated in 2975 RA patients (22). TA increases were seen in 12%, 16%, 19% and 14%, and neutropenia in 2.3%, 5.5%, 3.9% and 4.2%. Pneumonitis played no role, with only five cases in the overall series. There is no other study of a similar size on the safety of this therapy.

Despite the lack of studies, the combination MTX + LEF remains the most commonly used csDMARD combination therapy in Germany (23). However, to date there is no clear statement regarding the slowing of radiological progression. The toxicity risk of the combination, which was initially viewed critically and led to the classification of both substances as 'not recommended' in the product information, appears to be rather manageable based on current experience and the data presented above. Nevertheless, reliable monitoring with regular laboratory tests, in particular the TAs, is necessary.

4.2.2. Triple combination MTX + SSZ + HCQ (O'Dell regimen)

Internationally, this triple combination therapy, which continues to play a minor role in Germany, is by far the most commonly used csDMARD combination therapy. It goes back to two studies conducted by James O'Dell as first author (24, 25). In the first, 102 patients (average duration of illness approx. eight years) with insufficient response to at least one DMARD (including MTX in 11 cases) were randomly treated with MTX (starting with 7.5 mg per week, increase to 17.5 mg possible), SSZ (2 × 500 mg) + HCQ (2 × 200 mg) or the combination of the three substances for two years. An improvement of at least 50% in the modified Paulus criteria (no longer used as an outcome parameter) was the primary endpoint of the study, which was achieved significantly more often with the triple combination (77%) than with MTX (33%) and SSZ + HCQ (40%). The SJC decreased from 31 to 5 with MTX, from 31 to 7 with SSZ + HCQ and from 27 to 2 with the triple combination, with the groups differing significantly less. Radiology and functional status were not recorded.

This also applied to the follow-up study, which was completed over two years with 171 patients. The triple combination was randomized and compared with the combinations MTX + SSZ and MTX + HCQ. MTX was administered orally in doses ranging from 7.5 mg at the start to 17.5 mg. SSZ was administered twice a day, increasing to 1000 mg twice a day, and HCQ was administered twice a day. Many patients had already responded inadequately to MTX before the study, which led to significantly better results in the MTX-naive patients. In this study, too, the triple combination performed better than MTX + SSZ and MTX + HCQ, with ACR20 and ACR50 responses being 78/49/60% and 55/29/40%, respectively. Only 14/171 patients discontinued treatment prematurely due to adverse effects, which were equally distributed between the groups.

In the FIN-RACo study, 199 patients with early RA (<2 years of disease duration) were randomized, but with an open design, to be treated for two years with either triple therapy (MTX up to 15 mg per week, SSZ up to 2 g daily, HCQ 300 mg daily) or with SSZ monotherapy (up to 3 g daily), a comparator therapy that is not entirely adequate from today's perspective, but which could be replaced by MTX in case of non-response after six months (26). Intra-articular administration of GC was permitted, as was oral administration of 5 mg prednisolone with optional increase to 7.5 mg after three months. Against this background, high response rates were found, each with a significant advantage for the combination (ACR remission 37 vs 18%, ACR50 response 71 vs 58%), the GC requirement (oral and intraarticular) was higher in the monotherapy group. Radiologically, there was minimal progression in the combination group and significant progression in the monotherapy group. There was no difference in toxicity (against the background of an unusually high dose in the SSZ monotherapy group). Long-term radiological data over 11 years were available for 65 patients from each group (27). During this time, the LARSEN score increased by 17 points in the combination group and by 27 points in the monotherapy group; 87 and 72%, respectively, remained without erosive changes in the large joints.

In a randomized, single-blind, controlled British study, 96 patients with early RA without prior SSZ or MTX therapy were compared with primary triple therapy over one year with a step-up approach (SSZ 40 mg/kg daily ⇒ + MTX 7.5 mg per week, as required up to 25 mg per week ⇒ HCQ 400 mg daily, increasing if LDA was not achieved) (28). A good clinical response was achieved in both groups without significant differences (examples: DAS remission 33 vs 45%, ACR70 response 20 vs 30%), as well as a slight radiological progression that was comparable in both groups (6.6 vs 6.0). The good efficacy was offset by a high rate of AEs and 15/49 and 17/47 AE-related discontinuations, respectively.

A recent single-blind, randomized one-year study (tREACH) in 281 MTX-naive patients with early RA compared triple therapy in combination with intramuscular GC (group 1) and in combination with oral GC (start 15 mg, dose reduction, group 2) with a third group with MTX mono + GC as in group 2 (29). In this study, high doses (25 mg MTX per week orally, SSZ 2 g per day, HCQ 400 mg per day) were used. If LDA was not achieved, therapy could be intensified with biologics (etanercept (ETA), adalimumab (ADA), abatacept (ABC)) and reduced in two consecutive visits if remission occurred. The groups 1 and 2 offered a better clinical response, but the differences were not large: The DAS improved in all three groups by 1.8, 1.8 and 1.7, the HAQ by 0.5, 0.4 and 0.5, a DAS remission was achieved by 61, 54 and 51%, and a Boolean remission by 22, 16 and 16%. Radiologically, no differences were seen. Biologics were required more frequently in the MTX group (43%) than in the two triple groups (29 and 26% respectively). In the two triple groups, however, treatment discontinuations were significantly more frequent than in the MTX group. Further studies including triple therapy were carried out with biologics and are presented in the relevant chapter.

Adherence problems are rarely recorded in time-limited RCTs. In our own patient population, triple therapy is rarely tolerated, and premature termination of SSZ therapy in particular is the rule. According to numerous colleagues, this seems to be a widespread problem, at least in Germany. Against this background, it is not surprising that in the last available evaluation of the DRFZ's "Kerndokumentation" data from 2019 (23), not only has the general proportion of csDMARD combination therapies declined sharply to 6%, but within this group triple therapy only plays a minor role with a share of less than 2%. International long-term studies also show significant adherence problems with triple therapy. In the evaluation of an American insurance database, 3724 combination therapies ETA + MTX were retrospectively compared with 818 triple therapies over several years (30). Adherence after one year was significantly lower with triple therapy at 18% vs 28%.

The benefits of the triple combination therapy MTX + SSZ + HCQ have now been sufficiently proven by studies, including comparative studies with biologics, which are discussed elsewhere. There is no head-to-head comparison with the second widely used csDMARD combination MTX + LEF. However, due to the high demands on the patient (6 tablets daily in addition to MTX) and the increased rate of adverse effects, this combination is rarely used in Germany.

4.2.3. Combinations MTX + SSZ and MTX + HCQ / MTX + CQ

In addition to the experience from the second O'Dell study (see above), in which the triple combination proved to be superior to MTX + SSZ and MTX + HCQ, the combination MTX + SSZ in particular has been tested several times in a controlled manner. An RCT examined this combination in 105 previously untreated patients with early RA over 52 weeks in comparison to the individual substances; the dosage for SSZ was 2000 (up to 3000) mg, for MTX 7.5 (up to 15) mg per week (31). There was an improvement in all three groups, but the differences were not significant – this against the background that most patients were underdosed by today's standards in the MTX monotherapy group. The dropout rate in the combination group was significantly higher than in the MTX monotherapy group. A second study with identical design, identical initial population and identical dosages was conducted in 209 patients (32). Here, too, the improvement rate in the three groups – as well as the radiological progression rate – was not different (e.g. ACR20 response 59/59/65%), but the rate of adverse events was significantly increased in the combination group.

In the randomized controlled MASCOT study, MTX + SSZ and MTX monotherapy or SSZ monotherapy (combined with placebo) were compared in 165 SSZ-pretreated RA patients with an average disease duration of one year (33). The combination was superior to the individual substances, but the improvement rates were overall in a surprisingly low range (remission at 10/3/5%, ACR20/50/70 response at 29/11/4% vs 15/7/2% vs 18/6/2%). Here, too, the discontinuation rates were rather high at 17/56, 14/55 and 16/54.

When used in combination with MTX, HCQ significantly increases its AUC, as shown in a randomized crossover study (34). Despite this possible advantage of the combination, the good clinical effects of the MTX + HCQ combination found in the second O'Dell study (see above) could not be confirmed by a second study. The MTX + HCQ combination was studied in a controlled manner with MTX monotherapy (dose only 7.5 mg per week) in Brazil in 82 RA patients (35). Joint count, grip strength and functional limitation were measured as efficacy parameters, with advantages for the combination in each case. The surprising result of the comparison MTX + LEF vs MTX + HCQ (see above) also deserves mention. A recent Chinese study with a controlled comparison between the TCM treatment *Qingre Huoxue* and the combination MTX + HCQ in 468 patients (36). The ACR20/50/70 response under TCM, MTX+HCQ combination and combination of both procedures was 73 vs 80 vs 74%, 41 vs 48 vs 51% and 21 vs 22 vs 25%, the differences were not significant. The AE rate was significantly lower under TCM.

Overall, the data on the benefit of the combinations MTX + SSZ and MTX + HCQ appear to be rather limited; to date there is no evidence of any added value compared to optimized MTX monotherapy (administered parenterally, dosed at the upper limit). In addition, there is no evidence at all of any effect inhibiting destruction. Furthermore, in the case of the combination MTX + SSZ, there is an obvious adherence problem, probably due to low tolerability and the number of tablets taken daily. In view of the many effective alternatives, these combinations therefore seem unnecessary from today's perspective.

4.2.4. Studies using the COBRA regimen

The COBRA regimen developed in Holland uses a combination of MTX (only 7.5 mg per week) + SSZ (2000 g per day), and an initial dose of 60 mg prednisolone, which is then rapidly reduced. Similar to the FIN-RACo study (see above), the original COBRA study (37) used SSZ monotherapy as a comparison. As expected, the combination was clearly superior after 28 weeks (examples ACR20 72 vs 49%, ACR50 49 vs 27%). An evaluation of the long-term course 11 years after the study still showed advantages for the original combination group in terms of radiological progression, but a higher prevalence of hypertension, diabetes mellitus and cataracts in this group (38).

In addition to the use of SSZ as a control, the arbitrary choice of an extremely high corticosteroid starting dose was a major criticism of this study. In fact, another open, randomized controlled study comparing the COBRA regimen with a COBRA "light" combination (starting dose 30 instead of 60 mg prednisolone, MTX escalation up to 25 mg per week possible, without SSZ) over six months offered largely similar results in both groups, such as minimal disease activity in 49 vs 41% (39). More recently, the CARERA study in patients with early RA randomized the classic COBRA regimen to compare the combination MTX + 30 mg prednisone (with rapid GC dose reduction) and the combination MTX + LEF + 30 mg prednisone (with rapid GC dose reduction) (40). After 16 weeks, the three groups did not differ in efficacy, but the MTX+prednisone group had significantly fewer treatment-related adverse events (47 vs 61 and 69%, respectively).

The selection of studies presented here is not complete: In some strategy studies, MTX combinations with other DMARDs represent only one of many steps in the algorithm, which makes an exact assessment of the individual combinations difficult (BeST study), or the primary objective of the study was the strategy and not the value of the individual combinations used (TICORA, CAMERA study). These studies are therefore not discussed in detail here.

> The COBRA study was the first to show the large benefit of a combination with integrated step-down GC administration. However, from today's perspective, the classic COBRA regimen seems outdated due to the high GC starting dose; using 30 mg (possibly even 20 mg) instead of 60 mg appears to be equally effective. According to the results of the CARERA study, starting RA therapy with MTX + step-down GC is as effective as a csDMARD combination with MTX, but better tolerated. The EULAR Recommendations and the German S2 guideline have also adopted this approach.

4.3. Studies on the combination of methotrexate + TNF inhibitors

TNF-α inhibitors generally work better in combination with MTX than in monotherapy. ETA performs somewhat better in monotherapy than the other substances in the group, but should also be used in combination if possible. Infliximab (INX) and golimumab (GLM) are generally only approved for combination therapy (in RA).

4.3.1. Infliximab

The combination INX + MTX was investigated in two large studies, ATTRACT and ASPIRE, in advanced and early RA (41, 42). The most important results of both studies are shown in Table 4.1. In the ATTRACT study, the control group consisted of patients who had previously not responded adequately to MTX and whose inadequate treatment was now continued, which limits the significance of the comparison. Despite advanced, highly active disease, the study showed complete elimination of radiological progression with the combination as the most important result, while the clinical response rates were rather moderate by today's standards (e.g. ACR70 response 8%), probably due to the characteristics of the patient population.

The ASPIRE study, on the other hand, was conducted in cases of highly active but early RA. Considering the *de novo* therapy in the three treatment groups (MTX + placebo vs MTX + INX 3 mg/kg vs MTX + INX 6 mg/kg), a fair comparison can be assumed here. Clinically, the 3 mg group offered significantly better results in many parameters compared to MTX mono, but the difference was surprisingly small (example: DAS28 remission 21 vs 15%). The 6 mg/kg group performed better overall (example: DAS28 remission 31%). This study also confirmed the ability of the INX + MTX combination to almost completely suppress radiological progression. This effect was also observed in the combination in patients who clinically showed a rather moderate response, but this did not apply to the MTX monotherapy group (43). In the START study, the ATTRACT results were later confirmed with even slightly better results (also in patients with advanced disease) (☞ Table 4.1) – it is noteworthy that no better results were achieved with 10 mg/kg IFX than with 3 mg/kg (44). A num-

Study (Ref.)	Patients/ duration of disease	Duration of study	Comparison	ACR20/50/70 response (%)	DAS28 remission	Radiology (mTSS)
ATTRACT* (42)	516 ∅ 8-9 years MTX-IR patientes	30 weeks / 54 weeks (extension)	INX + MTX vs Placebo + MTX in MTX non-responders	50/27/8 vs 20/5/0	not assessed	+7.9 vs –0.66 (week 54)
ASPIRE* (43)	1,049 ∅ 9 months	12 moths	INX + MTX 3 mg/kg vs INX + MTX 6 mg/kg vs Placebo + MTX in *de novo* therapy	62/46/33 vs 66/50/37 vs 54/32/21	21% vs 31% vs 15%	+0.4 vs +0.5 vs +3.7
START (45)	1,084 6-8 years	22 weeks	INX + MTX 3 mg/kg vs INX + MTX 10 mg/kg vs Placebo + MTX in MTX non-responders	58/32/14 vs 61/35/16 vs 26/10/5	31% vs 32% vs 14%	not assessed

Table 4.1: Examples of combination studies INX + MTX. **mTSS**: modified Total Sharp Score.
* The ATTRACT study shows the results for the approval dosage of INX (3 mg/kg every eight weeks), the ASPIRE study shows the results for 3 mg/kg and 6 mg/kg (approved retrospectively).

ber of other smaller INX combination studies with a similar design did not lead to any new findings.

In the Swedish SWEFOT study, the combination MTX + INX was compared with the triple combination MTX + SSZ + HCQ in patients with early RA who had not previously achieved LDA with MTX (45). One year after the start of the study, the combination MTX + INX showed clinically significant advantages (examples of primary outcome parameters EULAR good response 39 vs 25%, ACR70 response 28 vs 15%). After two years, however, there was no longer any clinical difference between the two combinations (46). Radiologically, the combination MTX + INX was significantly superior both after one and two years.

In the NEO-RACo study, patients with very early, DMARD-naive RA were treated for four weeks with MTX + SSZ + HCQ and a fixed dose of 7.5 mg prednisolone. and permitted intraarticular administration of prednisolone, then randomized to INX 3 mg/kg or placebo (47). Clinically, there were no significant differences between the two groups, with an overall excellent response (e.g. DAS28 remission 82% in each case). The INX combination performed significantly better in terms of the radiological score (no progression) and the proportion of patients with remission lasting over two years (72% vs 49%).

INX is only approved for RA therapy in combination with MTX, so a comparison with INX monotherapy is neither possible nor meaningful. The combination has been established for many years, and radiological changes or progression can be almost completely prevented. In a direct comparison in patients with early RA, the triple combination MTX + SSZ + HCQ appears to be clinically almost equivalent to the combination MTX + INX – especially when optimized by concomitant corticoid therapy.

4.3.2. Etanercept

In contrast to INX, ETA is approved for both monotherapy and combination with MTX. In the TEMPO study, the effectivity of monotherapy was initially compared with the combination over a period of one year, and MTX monotherapy was also compared in a third arm (48). The most important one-year results of this study can be found in Table 4.2. All groups showed good therapeutic success. The combination performed significantly better than both monotherapies in all parameters, with ETA only numerically being slightly more effective than MTX in the latter. Radiologically, there was slight progression with MTX monotherapy, and a standstill in both other groups. These results were confirmed in the second year of treatment (49), where it was found that the discontinuation rate in the combination therapy was also significantly lower at 29% (vs 39% ETA monotherapy and 48% MTX monotherapy). In an open follow-up study following the TEMPO study, which ran for a total of three years, the patients previously treated with monotherapy were treated with the combination for 52 weeks, i.e. the ETA monotherapy group received MTX, and the MTX monotherapy group received ETA (50). The results confirmed the superiority of the combination: the proportion of patients in DAS remission increased significantly from 24 to 42% in the MTX ⇒ MTX + ETA group, and non-significantly from 27 to 37% in the ETA ⇒ ETA + MTX group.

The prospective randomized open Japanese JESMR study confirmed the advantage of the ETA + MTX combination compared to ETA monotherapy with a different study approach: patients with insufficient MTX response were treated with ETA, and MTX therapy was randomly continued or omitted for 52 weeks (51). The ACR20/50/70 response was 86/77/51% with the combination, 64/44/29% with ETA monotherapy, and the DAS28 remission was 36 vs 19%. The proportion of patients without radiological progression was 57 vs 40%.

Omitting MTX after long-term ETA+ MTX combination therapy is not always successful: in the CAMEO study, patients were randomly assigned to continue treatment with the combination or ETA monotherapy after six months of combination therapy (52). In patients with LDA status at the time of randomization, this status was maintained after a further six months in both groups. Patients with worse control after six months continued to improve over the next six months with the combination, but in patients treated with ETA monotherapy, disease activity increased again.

Analogous to ASPIRE with INX, a combination study was also conducted for ETA in early, active RA with MTX and ETA-naive patients: In the COMET study, MTX + ETA and MTX + placebo were compared in the first year of treatment (53). In all parameters, the combination proved to be superior with very good results (including DAS28 remission 50 vs 28%) (☞ Table 4.2). In the second year of treatment, the patients in the combination group were randomized to (continued) combination therapy or ETA monotherapy, while those in the MTX group were randomized to the combination or continued to receive MTX monotherapy (54). After two years, DAS38 remission remained higher with combination therapy at 57% compared to patients treated with ETA monotherapy (50%); in the original MTX group it was 58% (combination) and 35% (MTX continued mono). The proportion of patients without radiological progression was 90/75/75/67%. In summary, the COMET data also indicate advantages of the combination compared to both MTX monotherapy and (to a lesser extent) ETA monotherapy.

Like the SWEFOT study with INX, some comparative studies of triple therapy vs ETA + MTX, which, however, had methodological problems, show that an *a priori* combination of TNF blocker + MTX is not necessarily superior to DMARD combinations. As an example, in the RACAT study, which received a lot of attention in the USA, 353 patients with inadequate MTX response were randomized to ETA + MTX vs MTX + SSZ + HCQ for 24 weeks, and then switched for a further 24 weeks if there was no effect (55). The authors concluded that both therapies were equivalent, although ETA + MTX showed numerical advantages in almost all parameters after 26 weeks (ACR50/70 response 36/16% vs 25/5%, DAS-LDA 35 vs 25%, mTSS 0.003 vs 0.42, DAS28 improvement 2.1 vs 1.8). This is important in light of the significant methodological deficiencies: the primary endpoint was changed during the study. The estimated number of 450 patients required for full power was greatly undercut with 353 patients included, of whom only 309 had complete data, which probably prevented the differences from being significant. Despite the methodological weaknesses, this study confirms the value of MTX combination therapy in one form or another with overall good outcome data.

In contrast to INX, ETA can be used both as monotherapy and in combination with MTX. The majority of study results suggest that the combination ETA + MTX has advantages over ETA monotherapy, although monotherapy also leads to good results. A head-to-head comparison regarding the benefits of combination therapy does not exist for the five approved TNF inhibitors, including all biosimilars, so ETA + MTX can be considered a comparably effective therapy like combinations with other TNF blockers.

4.3.3. Adalimumab

Adalimumab (ADA) is also approved for monotherapy and in combination with MTX. The relation of the potency of both forms of administration was investigated in a randomized controlled study over two years in patients with early RA in the PREMIER study with MTX monotherapy as another comparison group (56). The combination was shown to be significantly superior to the monotherapies in all parameters including radiology and offered improvement rates that corresponded to those of comparable studies with other TNF inhibitors (e.g. COMET) (☞ also Table 4.2). The two monotherapies only differed radiologically, with ADA mono having clear advantages over MTX mono. The option of increasing the ADA dose to weekly administration if the ACR20 response was not achieved after week 16, was used by 11% vs 25% vs 20%. Following the RCT phase, the patients were followed for a further eight years in an open long-term extension study, meaning that 50% of the original RCT population could be followed for ten years (57). In these patients, the success was maintained over the entire period, including largely preventing radiological progression. The initial advantage of the combination therapy compared to monotherapies was maintained over the entire period, although mono group particpants were switched to the combination after two years and from then on, with an annualized increase in the mTSS of 0.48 and 0.58 between years 3 and 10, they no longer differed from the initial combination group (0.46).

In a head-to-head study, the combination ADA + MTX was compared with the combination ABC + MTX; the results can be found in the abatacept chapter.

According to the PREMIER data, ADA should certainly be used in combination with MTX if possible, but the MTX dose required was unclear for a long time. This question was investigated in the CONCERTO study: In 395 biologics- and MTX-naive patients with early RA, ADA was combined with 2.5 vs 5 vs 10 vs 20 mg MTX weekly in a randomized controlled trial over 26 weeks (58). Numerically, there was an increase in effect with increasing dose, but there was no longer any relevant difference between 10 and 20 mg (for example, the achievement of an LDA – corresponding to the primary endpoint – in 43, 44, 57 and 60% of patients). 10 mg weekly should therefore be a sufficient MTX dose when combined with TNF inhibitors, possibly also when combined with other biologics, but this has not yet been proven in studies.

An additional benefit of the combination partner MTX for ADA and the other TNF inhibitors is an improvement in long-term drug survival, as has been shown in several studies (59, 60). In an evaluation from the Italian GRISEA registry, the odds ratio for drug survival of TNF blocker therapy over four years was increased by 40% when combined with MTX.

Although ADA is approved for monotherapy, studies have shown that the combination with MTX is significantly more effective. To date, the longest study data for ADA + MTX with evidence of sustained good effectivity are available from the long-term results of the PREMIER study. As with the other TNF inhibitors, the combination with MTX significantly increases the prospects for good long-term drug survival. According to the data from the CONCERTO study, the required MTX dose in the combination is likely to be 10 mg per week. MTX can therefore be dosed at significantly lower doses in combination than previously in monotherapy or in combination with conventional DMARDs.

4.3.4. Certolizumab pegol and golimumab

Of the two most recently approved TNF inhibitors, certolizumab pegol (CZP) is approved for combination and monotherapy, whereas GLM is only approved for combination therapy with MTX. The relevant approval studies for CZP, RAPID 1 and 2 (61, 62), were carried out with the combination CZP + MTX vs MTX + placebo. Details of these studies can be found in Table 4.2. Both studies can be considered together, as they only differed from each other in terms of the duration of the study and partly in the form of administration. In both studies, the extent of clinical efficacy appears to be somewhat lower than in other TNF studies (☞ Table 4.2), which could be explained by the very high disease activity (DAS28 average 6.8) and long disease duration, as well as the rather low MTX dose used (average 12.2-12.6 mg per week). The radiological progression, which tends towards zero, is in line with other studies conducted with this mode of action. The response rates in the MTX

Study Drug (Ref.)	Patients/ disease duration	Study duration	Comparison	ACR20-/50-/70 response (%)	DAS/DAS28 remission (ESR)	Radiology (mTSS)
TEMPO ETA 1-year data (49)	682 ∅ 6-7 yrs	52 wks (later extension)	ETA + MTX vs ETA + placebo vs MTX + placebo in MTX-naive patients	85/69/43 vs 76/48/24 vs 75/43/19	35% vs 16% vs 13% (DAS <1.6)	–0.54 vs 0.52 vs +2.80
COMET ETA 1-year data (55)	542 ∅ 8-9 mo.	12 mo. (later extension)	ETA + MTX vs MTX + placebo in MTX-naive patients	86/71/48 vs 67/49/28	50% vs 28%	+0.27 vs +2.44
PREMIER ADA (60)	799 ∅ 8-9 mo.	24 mo.	ADA + MTX vs ADA mono vs MTX mono in MTX-naive patients	69/59/47 vs 49/37/28 vs 56/43/28	49% vs 25% vs 15%	+1.9 vs +5.5 vs +10.4
RAPID 1 CZP (65)	982 6.2 yrs MTX-IR patients	12 mo.	2 : 2 : 1 CZP 40 wks 0/2/4, then 200 mg 2w + MTX vs 400 mg 2w + MTX vs MTX + placebo	58.8/37.1/21.4 vs 60.8/39.9/20.6 vs 13.6/7.6/3.0	not assessed	+0,7 (both dosages) vs +3.0
RAPID 2 CZP (66)	619 5.6-6.5 yrs MTX-IR patients	6 mo.	like RAPID 1	57.3/32.5/15.9 vs 57.6/33.1/10.6 vs 8.7/3.1/0.8	9.4% vs 8.5% vs 0.8%	+0.2 vs –0.4 vs +1.2
GO-BEFORE GLM (69)	637 2.9-4.1 yrs	6 mo.	GLM 50 + MTX vs GLM 100 + MTX vs GLM 100 + placebo vs MTX + placebo	ACR20: 61.6/61.6/51.6/49.4 ACR50: 40.3/36.5/32.7/29.4 ACR70: 23.9/18.2/13.8/15.6	25.2% vs 19.5% vs 15.7% vs 11.3%	+0.74 vs +0.07 vs +1.25 vs +1.37 (week 52)

Table 4.2: Examples of combination studies MTX + ETA/+ ADA/+ CZP/+ GLM. **MTX-IR**: inadequate response to MTX; **mTSS**: modified Total Sharp Score.

control groups were extremely low (e.g. ACR50 response 7.6% in RAPID-1, 3.1% in RAPID-2), which can be explained by the design with MTX-IR patients.

Some studies have shown that CZP mono is effective, and it is therefore approved. Unfortunately, a controlled comparison of CZP + MTX vs CZP + placebo was not carried out. In REALISTIC, a randomized phase IIIb study, a real-life population of 1063 RA patients who received CZP in combination with MTX or (in smaller numbers) with other csDMARDs and in about 20% monotherapy, were initially treated for 12 weeks in a placebo-controlled manner (63), then openly in a 28-week extension study (64). Around 38% had already received TNF inhibitors. Only this study allows (uncontrolled) comparison of the combination of CZP + MTX and CZP + other csDMARDs with CZP monotherapy. The combination proved to be numerically more effective (no information on significance calculations), as in the ACR20/5070 response after 28 weeks (62/38/20% vs 48/27/11%).

The efficacy of GLM in combination with MTX was tested in three RCTs with different starting situations: GO-BEFORE (MTX-naive patients), GO-FORWARD (patients with inadequate response to MTX) and GO-AFTER (failure of at least one prior anti-TNF therapy). In all three studies, GLM offered significantly better results than the control group with MTX + placebo. As an example, Table 4.2 shows the results of the GO-BEFORE study (65), for which radiological data (66) and five-year results of the long-term extension (67) are also available. This study also included a GLM mono group with 100 mg every four weeks, which allows comparison with the combination (☞ Table 4.2). Clinically, the two GLM doses in combination with MTX proved to be significantly superior to the two monotherapy groups. These, in turn, did not differ from MTX + placebo in any parameter, i.e. similar to ADA monotherapy in the PREMIER study, GLM monotherapy in *de novo* therapy also appears to offer little clinical advantage over MTX, whereas the combination therapy is superior. Radiologically, the combination groups performed significantly better, but there was generally a very low progression rate (even after 52 weeks). More than two thirds of the patients on combination therapy with two GLM doses were still available for the five-year evaluation and offered very good clinical and radiological results (progression in the mTSS only 1.36!).

In terms of effectivity, CZP and GLM are generally similar to the other three TNF inhibitors. GLM is only approved for combination therapy with MTX, which also appears to be superior to monotherapy according to the results of GO-BEFORE. CZP can also be used as monotherapy. There is no RCT comparison of CZP + MTX vs CZP + placebo, but according to the results of the REALISTIC study, the combination should also have advantages compared to CZP monotherapy, so CZP should also be used in combination with MTX if possible.

4.4. Studies on the combination of methotrexate with non-TNF biologics

- + Abatacept (ABC)
- + Rituximab (RTX)
- + Tocilizumab (TCZ)
- + Sarilumab (SAR)
- + Anakinra

From a large number of existing studies on the combination of ABC, RTX and TCZ with MTX, a few representative studies are presented in more detail below; for a complete overview, please refer to the relevant reviews.

Abatacept

Abatacept is only approved for the treatment of RA in combination with MTX. The combination was shown to be effective in advanced RA in the AIM study (68, 69) in patients with inadequate response to MTX, and in the ATTAIN study (70) in patients previously treated with anti-TNF. The results of the AIM study are shown as examples in Table 4.3. ABC + MTX was clinically clearly superior to MTX monotherapy, albeit in a population that had previously responded inadequately to MTX. Radiologically, an overall low progression was also noted, which is also an advantage for the combination. The long-term extension over five years was completed by 72% of patients with a sustained good response (DAS28 remission 25%), which confirms a very good drug survival rate (71). Radiologically, the mTSS only increased by 2.2 points during this period.

In the AVERT study, the combination was randomized to compare with ABC + placebo and MTX + placebo in patients with early RA (72). In this phase IIIb study, ABC was administered subcutaneously, in contrast to the early studies. The most important AVERT results can also be found in Table 4.3. This study is particularly important because, under modern methodological conditions, the superiority of the ABC + MTX combination compared to ABC monotherapy could be confirmed, and ABC monotherapy was not more effective than MTX monotherapy. Finally, in AMPLE, one of the few biologics studies with a head-to-head design available to date, the ABC +

Study Drug (Ref.)	Patients/ disease duration	Study duration	Comparison	ACR20/50/70 response (%)	DAS/DAS28 remission (ESR)	Radiology (mTSS)
AIM ABC (72)	652 ∅ 8-9 yrs MTX-IR pat.	52 wks (later extension)	ABC + MTX vs MTX + Placebo	73.1/48.3/28.8 vs 39.7/18.2/6.1	not assessed	+1.21 vs +2.32
AVERT ABC (76)	511 ∅ 6-7 mo.	12 mo. (later extension with weaning)	ABC + MTX vs ABC + placebo vs MTX + placebo	74.8/63/52.1 vs 65.5/53.4/38.8 vs 63.8/46.6/34.5	60.9% vs 42.5% vs 45.2%	no X-rays
SERENE RTX (78)	511 ∅ 7 yrs MTX-IR pat.	24 wks with extension till wk. 48	RTX 2× 500 mg + MTX vs RTX 2× 1,000 mg + MTX vs Placebo + MTX	54.5/26.3/9 vs 50.6/25.9/10.9 vs 23.3/9.3/5.2%	9.4% vs 9.6% vs 2.3%	not assessed
IMAGE RTX (79)	755 ∅ 11 mo.	12 mo.	RTX 2× 500 mg + MTX vs RTX 2× 1.00, mg + MTX vs Placebo + MTX	77/59/42 vs 80/65/47 vs 64/42/25	25% vs 31% vs 13%	+0.64 vs +0.36 vs +1.08
LITHE TCZ (83)	1196 9-9.5 yrs MTX-IR pat.	12 mo. with extension by further 12 mo.	TCZ 8 mg/kg + MTX vs TCZ 4 mg/kg + MTX vs Placebo + MTX	54/33/19 vs 47/31/14 vs 23/9/3	47.2% vs 30.2% vs 7.9%	+0.29 vs +0.34 vs +1.13
ACT-RAY TCZ (87)	556 8.2-8.3 yrs MTX-IR pat.	6 mo. with extension to 2 yrs	TCZ 8 mg/kg + MTX vs TCZ 8 mg/kg + placebo	71.5/45.5/24.5 vs 70.3/40.2/25.4	40.4% vs 34.8%	+0.08 vs +0.22
MOBILTY	1197 8.6-9.5 yrs MTX-IR pat.	52 wks	SAR 200 + MTX SAR150 + MTX Placebo + MTX	59/43/27% 54/40/25% 32/18/9%	34.1 vs 31.0 vs 8.5%	0.25 vs 0.90 vs 2.78
TARGET	546 11.6-12.7 yrs TNF-IR pat.	24 wks	SAR 200 + MTX SAR150 + MTX Placebo + MTX	60.9/40.8/16.3% 55.8/37/19.9% 33.7/18.2/7.2%	28.8 vs 24.9 vs 7.2%	not assessed

Table 4.3: Examples of combination studies MTX + ABC/+ RTX/+ TCZ.
MTX-IR: inadequate response to MTX; **mTSS**: modified Total Sharp Score.

MTX combination was shown to be equally effective compared to the ADA + MTX combination in 646 patients with an average disease duration of almost two years. Here, too, ABC was administered subcutaneously (73).

ABC has proven to be equally effective as the TNF inhibitors under controlled conditions. It is only approved in combination with MTX, but the results of the AVERT study show that the combination also has clear advantages.

Rituximab

For RTX, too, there is only approval for combined use with MTX in RA. Among several controlled studies comparing the effect of the combination and MTX + placebo in patients with inadequate MTX response, SERENE is the largest and longest phase III study (74); its most important results are shown in Table 4.3. Two different RTX doses (2 × 500 vs 2 × 1000 mg) were compared with MTX and led to identical response rates that were significantly better than the control group. The particularly low improvement rates with MTX are also favored by the design (MTX-IR). As in other studies, the response also continued to increase after the second cycle in week 48. Seropositive patients offered higher response rates than seronegative ones.

MTX-naive patients were examined in the IMAGE study (75); here too, the main results can be found in Table 4.3. With a similar design but a much shorter duration of disease, this study found significantly higher response rates, which also included the inhibition of radiological progression. As in the SERENE study, seropositive patients showed a higher response than seronegative ones; the ACR70 response in the approved dosage was 50 vs 25%, and there was no significant difference in seronegativity between RTX + MTX and placebo + MTX. The difference between the RTX dosages 2 × 1000 mg and 2 × 500 mg was rather small.

RTX monotherapy compared to RTX + MTX has not been investigated in RCTs, but only in an early proof-of-concept study (76) and in a non-interventional study (77). In the former study with an open, randomized design, the combinations RTX + MTX and RTX + ciclophosphamide (CIP) proved to be superior primarily to MTX monotherapy, but to a lesser extent also to RTX monotherapy (example: ACR70 response after 48 weeks 35 vs 27 vs 5 vs 15%). In the non-interventional study conducted in Germany with 2484 patients, the response rates for RTX monotherapy were at a similar level to those for the combinations RTX + MTX and RTX + LEF. However, an analysis from the German RABBIT registry, which presumably includes some of the same patients, shows that drug survival under RTX monotherapy is significantly worse than under the combinations, with an HR of 1.7 for discontinuation (78).

RTX also offers an effectivity comparable to that of other biologics under controlled conditions. It is also only approved in combination with MTX. Unlike ABC, the effectiveness of the combination compared to monotherapy has not been investigated in RCTs, but according to the data mentioned above, the combination appears to have advantages regardless of the approval situation.

Tocilizumab

Tocilizumab (TCZ) is approved for both monotherapy and combination with MTX. In monotherapy, it shows better effectivity data than the other approved biologics; the data on TCZ monotherapy will not be discussed here. Some studies have compared the effectivity of the combination TCZ + MTX with MTX monotherapy and in some cases also with TCZ monotherapy. Choosing from a very broad range of studies, only some will be discussed in more detail here as examples.

In the LITHE study, patients with a previously inadequate response to MTX were treated in a randomized controlled trial with TCZ + MTX (TCZ in doses of 8 mg/kg vs 4 mg/kg) vs placebo + MTX, including radiological follow-up (79). In the published one-year data, the combination in both doses was clinically and radiologically significantly superior to MTX + placebo, with only a small numerical difference between the two doses. In this study, too, radiological progression was very low in all three treatment groups (see below for treatment safety). An overview of the most important results is provided in Table 4.3. Other phase III RCTs with a similar design (inclusion of patients with inadequate response to previous treatment with conventional DMARDs) led to similar clinical results with superiority of the TCZ+DMARD group compared to the placebo+DMARD group; radiological data were not collected here. In the TOWARD study with 1216 patients, approximately 75% of the patients were treated with the combination TCZ + MTX, 25% with TCZ in combination with other DMARDs for 24 weeks (80). As in LITHE study, the OPTION study, was conducted with patients who had previously not responded adequately to MTX, included data from 623 patients and also had a treatment duration of 24 weeks (81). RADIATE, a third 24-week RCT, was conducted in 499 patients with inadequate response to TNF blockers (82). In line with the patient population that had exhausted all other treatment options, the response rates here were somewhat lower (e.g. DAS28 remission 30% under 8 mg/kg, 8% under 4 mg/kg TCZ, 2% under placebo – each in combination with MTX), but with significant advantages of the combination TCZ + MTX.

ACT-RAY, another phase III RCT, compared TCZ + MTX with TCZ + placebo in 556 patients with inadequate response to MTX, including radiological data (83); the most important results of the 24-week evaluation are contained in Table 4.3. The clinical and radiological response was very good in both groups; the combination showed a slightly higher response rate numerically in some parameters, but no significant differences were found. The one-year data published later (84) showed an overall increase in clinical response and continued minimal radiological progression. In some parameters (e.g. DAS remission 46% vs 37%, proportion of patients without radiological progression 93% vs 86%), the difference between the MTX combination and monotherapy groups now reached a significant level. For the sake of completeness, it should be mentioned that the SUMMACTA study demonstrated equal efficacy when comparing intravenous and subcutaneous administration of TCZ in combination with MTX under controlled conditions (85). A study comparing TCZ + MTX vs TCZ monotherapy vs MTX monotherapy in MTX-naive patients with early RA has not been published in detail at the time of printing of this book.

In terms of safety, TCZ's rate of severe infections is roughly comparable to that of TNF inhibitors: in an analysis of 5 RCTs including extension phases, it was 4.5/100 patient years (86). A special feature of TCZ compared to other biologics is an increased rate of perforations in the lower intestinal sections: in an evaluation from the German RABBIT registry, this rate was 3.44 per 1000 patient years compared to 0.67 under csDMARD, 0.66 under ETA or 0.64 under ABC (87). Co-medication with GC increased the risk. A comparison of the safety between TCZ + MTX and TCZ monotherapy can be found primarily in the data from the ACT-RAY study (see above). In the evaluation of the entire study period of 104 weeks (88), the rates of AEs, SAEs and treatment discontinuations due to AEs did not differ between the two groups. The rate of severe infections was slightly higher with combination therapy at 4.4/100 patient years than with monotherapy at 2.7. Another difference was found in the liver values: an increase in transaminases of 1.5-3 times above normal was seen in 30 vs 17%, 3-5 times above normal in 10 vs 4% and more than five times above normal in 4 vs 1%.

TCZ shows better effectivity in monotherapy compared to the other biologics. However, according to data from some studies, the combination with MTX appears to offer slight advantages over monotherapy, so that the combination with MTX is also initially preferred for this biologic, provided there are no MTX contraindications or intolerances. In terms of therapeutic safety, however, there is a slightly higher rate of SIEs and elevated liver enzymes with the combination. According to current knowledge, intestinal perforations do not occur more frequently with the combination than with monotherapy.

Sarilumab

Sarilumab (SAR) is another IL-6 receptor (IL6R) inhibitor that has been available for the treatment of RA for several years and can be used in two doses (200 or 150 mg subcutaneously every two weeks). Similar to TCZ, SAR shows very good efficacy both in monotherapy and in combination with MTX; there is no H2H comparison between the use of monotherapy and combination therapy. The effectivity of the combination was investigated in one study each in patients with inadequate response to MTX (MOBILITY, 89) and inadequate response to TNF inhibitors (TARGET, 90). In MOBILITY, the proportion of patients in DAS28-CRP remission after 52 weeks was 34% (SAR 200),

31% (SAR 150) and 9% (placebo), and in CDAI remission it was 18%, 15% and 5%. Radiological progression in W52 was 0.3, 0.9 and 2.8 points in the total Sharp score. In TARGET, the extent of improvement was somewhat lower, not unexpectedly due to the more difficult patient population, with DAS28-CRP remission of 29% (SAR 200), 25% (SAR 150) and 7% (placebo) and CDAI remission of 8%, 9% and 5% after 24 weeks. In TARGET, a small proportion of patients used other csDMARDs as MTX combination partners for SAR. In all SAR studies, the safety profile was consistent with that of the other IL6R inhibitor TCZ.

Like TCZ, SAR offers better effectivity in monotherapy compared to other biologics. The combination with MTX has proven to be effective in several studies. There is no direct comparison between the effectivity of monotherapy and combination therapy – as with TCZ, the guidelines recommend that treatment should initially be carried out in combination with MTX. The safety profile corresponds to that of TCZ.

Anakinra

The interleukin-1 inhibitor Anakinra, which is also approved for the treatment of RA, but only in combination with MTX, has proven to be significantly less effective compared to the other biologics (91, 92). It is therefore de facto no longer used to treat RA today.

4.5. Studies on the combination of methotrexate with JAK inhibitors

- + Tofacitinib (TOF)
- + Baricitinib (BAR)
- + Upadacitinib (UPA)
- + Filgotinib (FIL)

A total of four substances from the group of JAK inhibitors are approved in Germany for the treatment of RA; they can be used in combination with MTX or as monotherapy. While the combination with TOF may have slight advantages over monotherapy (see below), monotherapy appears to be equivalent for the other three substances. The most important studies are summarized in Table 4.4.

Tofacitinib

In the ORAL STRATEGY study, TOF mono was compared with TOF + MTX and ADA + MTX in a controlled manner over one year (93). In this study, the combination proved to be somewhat more effective than monotherapy, but the differences were not very large (exact results ☞ Table 4.4). In contrast to the three other JAK inhibitors, which have a priori approval for monotherapy, TOF is only approved in monotherapy if MTX is not available as a combination partner.

Baricitinib

BAR monotherapy and combination therapies were compared primarily in the phase III RA BEGIN study (94), but its first-line use in this study does not correspond to the approval status. The comparison included MTX monotherapy in addition to BAR in the approved dosage as monotherapy and in combination. Monotherapy and combination therapies proved to be equally effective and were significantly superior to MTX monotherapy (exact results ☞ Table 4.4). Radiological progression was minimal in all three groups. In the long-term extension study RA BEYOND, patients from all three groups of this study were continued with monotherapy (95). Patients from both BAR groups, including BAR + MTX, maintained efficacy with monotherapy, while patients on MTX monotherapy benefited from switching to BAR monotherapy. However, a small group of patients with insufficient efficacy in the original study on BAR monotherapy experienced an improvement in status with the addition of MTX.

Upadacitinib

UPA has demonstrated good efficacy in a number of studies both in combination with MTX and as monotherapy. There is no study directly comparing these two regimes. In a comparative analysis of two phase III studies with comparable designs (SELECT-NEXT with combination, SELECT-MONOTHERAPY with UPA monotherapy), largely the same efficacy was found in a total of 1114 patients (96). The ACR20/50/70 response was 68/42/23% in the UPA approval dosage of 15 mg monotherapy and 66/41/21% in the combination. Remission was determined with DAS28-CRP at 28% vs 28%, with CDAI at 13% vs 10%.

Study (Ref.)	Patients/ disease duration	Study duration	Comparison	ACR20/50/70 response	DAS/DAS28 remission (BSG)	Radiology (mTSS)
ORAL STRATEGY TOF (93)	1146 Ø 5.4-6.1 yrs MTX-IR-Pat.	52 wks	TOF-Mono vs TOF + MTX vs ADL + MTX	62/39/21% vs 70/48/29% vs 68/45/26%	11% vs 15% vs 17%	not assessed
RA BEGIN (94)	588 Ø 1.3-1.9 yrs no or minimal csDMARD therapy	12 mo.	BAR-Mono vs BAR + MTX vs MTX-Mono	73/57/42% vs 73/62/46% vs 50/38/25%	25% vs 28% vs 16% (CDAI remission)	+0.25 vs +0.06 vs +0.21
FINCH 3 (97)	1249 1.9-2.6 yrs no or minimal MTX pre-treatment	52 wks	FIL 200 + MTX vs FIL 100 + MTX vs FIL 200-Mono vs MTX-Mono	62.3/47.8% vs 59.4/40.1% vs 61.4/45.2% vs 48.3/29.8% (ACR50/70 resp.)	34.9% vs 26.5% vs 26.2% vs 17.3% (CDAI remission)	not assessed

Table 4.4: Examples of comparative studies JAK inhibitors + MTX vs JAK inhibitor monotherapy.

Filgotinib

In the phase III FINCH 3 study, FIL in the two approved doses, each in combination with MTX, was compared with FIL 200 monotherapy and MTX monotherapy in patients with no or only very short prior MTX therapy (97). In this study, too, FIL + MTX and FIL monotherapy were equally effective and all three FIL groups were significantly superior to MTX (exact results ☞ Table 4.4). There were no significant differences between combination and monotherapy in terms of tolerability.

JAK inhibitors are a very effective therapy in combination with MTX. In contrast to bDMARDs, however, JAK inhibitors in monotherapy are just as effective as in combination with MTX, the only exception being TOF, with the combination being slightly more effective. The results from the RA BEYOND study, however, suggest that if monotherapy is not effective enough, the addition of MTX can bring about an improvement. There are no differences in tolerability of the four substances between monotherapy and combination therapy under study conditions.

4.6. References

1. Rau R. Kombinationen mit anderen Basistherapeutika. In: Das Methotrexat-Buch – Aktuelle Therapiekonzepte in der Rheumatologie und Dermatologie. UNI-MED Verlag 2007, Kap.10, 47-54.

2. McCarty DJ, Harman JG, Grassanovich JL et al. Combination drug therapy of seropositive rheumatoid arthritis. J Rheumatol 1995;22:1636-45.

3. Wilke WS, Scherrer YR, Clough JD. Combination chemotherapy for severe rheumatoid arthritis. Intern Med Specialist 1989;10:59-76.

4. Willkens RF, Sharp JT, Stablein DM et al. Comparison of azathioprine, methotrexate, and the combination of both in the treatment of rheumatoid arthritis. A 48 week controlled clinical trial with radiologic outcome assessment. Arthritis Rheum 1995;38:1799-1806.

5. Lee S, Solomon G. Combination D-penicillamine and methotrexate therapy: proposal for early and aggressive treatment for rheumatoid arthritis. Bull Hosp Jt Dis Orthop Inst 1990;50:160-168.

6. Ichikawa Y, Saito T, Yamanaka H et al. Therapeutic effects of the combination of methotrexate and bucillamine in early rheumatoid arthritis: a multicenter, double-blind, randomized controlled study. Mod Rheumatol 2005;15:323-328.

7. Williams HJ, Ward JR, Reading JC, et al. Comparison of auranofin, methotrxate, and the combination of both in the treatment of rheumatoid arthritis. Arthritis Rheum 1992;3:259-269.

8. Rau R, Schleusser B, Herborn G, Karger T. Longterm treatment of destructive rheumatoid arthritis with methotrexate. J Rheumatol 1997;24:1881-89.

9. Lehman AJ, Esdaile JM, Klinkhoff AV et al. A 48 week, randomized, double-blind, double-observer, placebo-controlled multicenter trial of combination methotrexate and intramuscular gold therapy in rheumatoid arthritis. Arthritis Rheum 2003;52:1360-1370.

10. Tugwell P, Pincus Z, Yocum D et al. Combination therapy with cyclosporine and methotrexate in severe rheumatoid arthritis. N Engl J Med 1995;333:137-141.

11. Stein CM, Pincus T, Yocum D et al. Combination treatment of severe rheumatoidarthritis with cyclosporine and methotrexate for forty-eight weeks: an open-label extension study. The Methotrexate-Cyclosporine Combination Study Group. Arthritis Rheum 1997;40: 1843-1851.

12. Gerards AH, Landewe RBM, Prins APA et al. Cyclosporin A monotherapy versus cyclosporin A and methotrexate combination therapy in patients with early rheumatoid arthritis: a double blind randomised placebo controlled trial. Ann Rheum Dis 2003;62:291-296.

13. Choy EH, Smith CM, Farewell V et al. Factorial randomised controlled trial of glucocorticoids and combination disease modifying drugs in early rheumatoid arthritis. Ann Rheum Dis 2008; 67:656–663.

14. Hetland ML, Stengaard-Pedersen K, Junker P et al. Combination treatment with methotrexate, cyclosporine, and intraarticular betamethasone compared with methotrexate and intraarticular betamethasone in early active rheumatoid arthritis: an investigator-initiated, multicenter, randomized, double-blind, parallel-group, placebo-controlled study. Arthritis Rheum 2066;54: 1401-1409.

15. Hetland ML, Stengaard-Pedersen K, Junker P et al. Radiographic progression and remission rates in early rheumatoid arthritis – MRI bone oedema and anti-CCP predicted radiographic progression in the 5-year extension of the double-blind randomised CIMESTRA trial. Ann Rheum Dis 2010; 69:1789-1795.

16. Kremer JM, Genovese MC, Cannon GW, et al. Concomitant leflunomide therapy in patients with active rheumatoid arthritis despite stable doses of methotrexate. A randomized, double-blind, placebo-controlled trial. Ann Intern Med 2002; 137:726.

17. Kremer J, Genovese M, Cannon GW et al. Combination leflunomide and methotrexate (MTX) therapy for patients with active rheumatoid arthritis failing MTX monotherapy: open-label extension of a randomized, double-blind, placebo controlled trial. J Rheumatol 2004;31:1521-1531.

18. Lee SS, Park YW, Park JJ et al. Combination treatment with leflunomide and methotrexate for patients with active rheumatoid arthritis.Scand J Rheumatol 2009;38:11-14.

19. Zhang L, Chen F, Geng S et al. Methotrexate (MTX) plus hydroxychloroquine versus MTX plus leflunomide in patients with MTX-resistant active rheumatoid arthritis: A 2-year cohort study in real world. J Inflamm Res 2020; 13:1141-1150.

20. FDA Drug Safety Communication: New boxed warning for severe liver injury with arthritis drug Arava (leflunomide). 2010, http://www.fda.gov/Drugs/DrugSafety/Postmarket-DrugSafetyInformationforPatientsandProviders/ucm218679.htm.

21. Savage RL. Leflunomide in combination therapy of rheumatoid arthritis. Drug Saf 2010;33:523-526.

22. Bird P, Griffiths H, Tymms K et al. The SMILE Study - safety of methotrexate in combination with leflunomide in rheumatoid arthritis. J Rheumatol 2013;40:228-235.

23. Deutsches Rheumaforschungszentrum, Daten der Kerndokumentation 2019, bisher unpubliziert.

24. O'Dell J, Haire C, Erickson N et al. Treatment of rheumatoid arthritis with methotrexate alone, sulfasalazine and hydroxychloroquine, or a combination of all three medications. N Engl J Med 1996;334:1287-1291.

25. O'Dell J. Leff R, Paulsen G et al. Treatment of rheumatoid arthritis with methotrexate and hydroxychloroquine, methotrexate and sulfasalazine, or a combination of the three medications. Arthritis Rheum 2002;46:1164-1170.

26. Möttönen T, Hannonen P, Leirisalo-Repo M et al. Comparison of combination therapy with single-drug therapy in early rheumatoid arthritis: a randomised trial. FIN-RACo trial group. Lancet 1999;353:1568-1573.

27. Rantalaiho V, Korpela M, Laasonen L et al. Early combination disease-modifying antirheumatic drug therapy and tight disease control improve long-term radiologic outcome in patients with early rheumatoid arthritis: the 11-year results of the Finnish Rheumatoid Arthritis Combination Therapy trial. Arthritis Res Ther 2010;12:R122.

28. Saunders SA, Capell HA, Stirling A et al. Triple therapy in early active rheumatoid arthritis. a randomized, single-blind, controlled trial comparing step-up and parallel treatment strategies. Arthritis Rheum 2008;58: 1310-1317.

29. De Jong PH, Hazes JM, Han HK et al. Randomised comparison of initial triple DMARD therapy with methotrexate monotherapy in combination with low-dose glucocorticoid bridging therapy; 1-year data of the tREACH trial. Ann Rheum Dis 2014;73:1331-1339.

30. Bonafede M, Johnson BH, Tang DH et al. Etanercept-methotrexate combination therapy initiators have greater adherence and persistence than triple therapy initiators with rheumatoid arthritis. Arthritis Care Res 2015.

31. Haagsma CJ, Blom HJ, Riel PL van et al. Combination of sulphasalazine and methotrexate versus the single components in early rheumatoid arthritis: a randomised, controlled, double-blind, 52 week clinical trial. Br J Rheumatol 1997; 36:1082-1088.

32. Dougados M, Combe B, CantagrelA et al. Combination therapy in early rheumatoid arthritis: a randomised, controlled, double blind 52 week clinical trial of sulphasalazine and methotrexate compared with the single components. Ann Rheum Dis 1999;58:220-225.

33. Capell HA, Madhok R, Porter DR et al. Combination therapy with sulfasalazine and methotrexate is more effective than either drug alone in patients with rheumatoid arthritis with a suboptimal response to sulfasalazine: results from the double- blind placebo-controlled MASCOT study. Ann Rheum Dis 2007;66:235-241.

34. Carmichael SJ, Beal J, Day RO, Tett SE. Combination therapy with methotrexate and hydroxychloroquine for rheumatoid arthritis increases exposure to methotrexate. J Rheumatol 2002;29:2077-2083.

35. Ferraz MB, Pinheiro GR, Helfenstein M, et al. Combination therapy with methotrexate and chloroquine in rheumatoid arthritis. A multicenter randomised placebo-controlled trial. Scand J Rheumatol 1994;23:231-236.

36.Gong X, Liu WX, Tang XP et al. Traditional Chinese Medicine Qingre Huoxue treatment vs. the combination of methotrexate and hydroxychloroquine for active rheumatoid arthritis: A multicenter, double-blind, randomized controlled trial. Front Pharmacol 2021;12.

37. Boers M, Verhoeven AC, Markusse HM, et al. Randomized comparison of combined step-down prednisolone, methotrexate and sulphasalazine with sulphasalazine alone in early rheumatoid arthritis. Lancet 1997; 350:309-318.

38. Van Tuyl LHD, Boers M, Lems WF et al. Survival, comorbidities and joint damage 11 years after the COBRA combination therapy trial in early rheumatoid arthritis. Ann Rheum Dis 2010;69:807-812.

39. Den Uyl D, ter Wee M, Boers M et al. A non-inferiority trial of an attenuated combination strategy ('COBRA-light') compared to the original COBRA strategy: clinical results after 26 weeks. Ann Rheum Dis 2014; 73:1071-1078.

40. Verschueren P, De Cock D, Corluy L et al. Methotrexate in combination with other DMARDs is not superior to methotrexate alone for remission induction with moderate-to-high-dose glucocorticoid bridging in early rheumatoid arthritis after 16 weeks of treatment: the CareRA trial. Ann Rheum Dis 2015;74:27-34.

41. Maini R, St Clair EW, Breedveld F et al. Infliximab (chimeric anti-tumour necrosis factor alpha monoclonal antibody) versus placebo in rheumatoid arthritis patients receiving concomitant methotrexate: a randomised phase III trial. ATTRACT Study Group. Lancet 1999;354:1932-1939.

42. St Clair EW, Heijde DM van der, Smolen JS et al. Combination of infliximab and methotrexate therapy for early rheumatoid arthritis: a randomized, controlled trial. Arthritis Rheum 2004;50:3432-3443.

44. Smolen JS, van der Heijde DMFM, St.Clair EW et al. Predictors of joint damage in patients with early rheumatoid arthritis treated with high-dose methotrexate with or without concomitant infliximab. Results From the ASPIRE Trial. Arthritis Rheum 2006;54:702-710.

45. Westhovens R, Yocum D, Han J et al. The safety of infliximab, combined with background treatments, among patients with rheumatoid arthritis and various comorbidities. Arthritis Rheum 2006;54:1075-1086.

45. Van Vollenhoven RF, Ernestam S, Geborek P et al. Addition of infliximab compared with addition of sulfasalazine and hydroxychloroquine to methotrexate in patients with early rheumatoid arthritis (Swefot trial): 1-year results of a randomised trial. Lancet 2009;374:459 - 466.

46. Van Vollenhoven RF, Geborek P, Forslind K et al. Conventional combination treatment versus biological treatment in methotrexate-refractory early rheumatoid arthritis: 2 year follow-up of the randomised, non-blinded, parallel-group Swefot trial. Lancet 2012;379:1712-1720.

47. Leirisalo-Repo M, Kautiainen H, Laasonen L et al. Infliximab for 6 months added on combination therapy in early rheumatoid arthritis: 2-year results from an investigator-initiated, randomised, double-blind, placebo-controlled study (the NEO-RACo Study). Ann Rheum Dis 2013;72:851-857.

48. Klareskog L, Heijde D van der, Jager JP de et al. Therapeutic effect of the combination of etanercept and methotrexate compared with each treatment alone in patients with rheumatoid arthritis: double-blind randomised controlled trial. Lancet 2004;363:675-681.

49. Van der Heijde D, Klareskog L, Rodriguez-Valverde V et al. Comparison of etanercept and methotrexate, alone and combined, in the treatment of rheumatoid arthritis. Two-year clinical and radiographic results from the TEMPO Study, a double-blind, randomized trial. Arthritis Rheum 2006;54: 1063-1074.

51. Van der Heijde D, Burmester G, Melo-Gomes J et al. The safety and efficacy of adding etanercept to methotrexate or methotrexate to etanercept in moderately active rheumatoid arthritis patients previously treated with monotherapy. Ann Rheum Dis 2008;67:182-188.

51. Kameda H, Kanbe K, Sato E et al. Continuation of methotrexate resulted in better clinical and radiographic outcomes than discontinuation upon starting etanercept in patients with rheumatoid arthritis: 52-week results from the JESMR Study. J Rheumatol 2011;38:1585-1592.

52. Pope JE, Haraoui B, Thorne JC et al. The Canadian methotrexate and etanercept outcome study: a randomised trial of discontinuing versus continuing methotrexate after 6 months of etanercept and methotrexate therapy in rheumatoid arthritis. Ann Rheum Dis 2014; 73:2144-2151.

53. Emery P, Breedveld FC, Hall S et al. Comparison of methotrexate monotherapy with a combination of methotrexate and etanercept in active, early, moderate to severe rheumatoid arthritis (COMET): a randomised, double-blind, parallel treatment trial. Lancet 2008;372: 375-382.

54. Emery P, Breedveld F, van der Heijde D et al. Two-year clinical and radiographic results with combination etanercept–methotrexate therapy versus monotherapy in early rheumatoid arthritis. Arthritis Rheum 2010;62: 674-682.

55. O'Dell JR, Mikuls TR, Taylor TH et al. Therapies for active rheumatoid arthritis after methotrexate failure. N Engl J Med 2013;369:307-318.

56. Breedveld FC, Weisman MH, Kavanaugh AF et al. The premier study a multicenter, randomized, double-blind clinical trial of combination therapy with adalimumab plus methotrexate versus methotrexate alone or adalimumab alone in patients with early, aggressive rheumatoid arthritis who had not had previous methotrexate treatment. Arthritis Rheum 2006;54:26-37.

57. Keystone EC, Breedveld FC, van der Heijde D et al. Longterm effect of delaying combination therapy with tumor necrosis factor inhibitor in patients with aggressive early rheumatoid arthritis: 10-year efficacy and safety of adalimumab from the randomized controlled PREMIER Trial with openlabel extension. J Rheumatol 2014;41:5-14.

58. Burmester GR, Kivitz AJ, Kupper H et al. Efficacy and safety of ascending methotrexate dose in combination with adalimumab: the randomised CONCERTO trial. Ann Rheum Dis 2015;74:1037-1044.

59. Soliman MM, Ashcroft DM, Watson KD et al. Impact of concomitant use of DMARDs on the persistence with anti-TNF therapies in patients with rheumatoid arthritis: Results from the British Society for Rheumatology Biologics Register. Ann Rheum Dis 2011;70:583-589.

60. Iannone F, Gremese E, Atzeni F et al. Longterm retention of tumor necrosis factor-α inhibitor therapy in a large Italian cohort of patients with rheumatoid arthritis from the GISEA Registry: An appraisal of predictors. J Rheumatol 2012;39: 1179-1184.

61. Keystone E, van der Heijde D, Mason Jr D et al. Certolizumab pegol plus methotrexate is significantly more effective than placebo plus methotrexate in active rheumatoid arthritis. Arthritis Rheum 2008;11:3319-3329.

62. Smolen J, Landewe RB, Mease P et al. Efficacy and safety of certolizumab pegol plus methotrexate in active rheumatoid arthritis: the RAPID 2 study. A randomised controlled trial. Ann Rheum Dis 2009;68:797-804.

63. Weinblatt ME, Fleischmann R, Huizinga TWJ et al. Efficacy and safety of certolizumab pegol in a broad population of patients with active rheumatoid arthritis: results from the REALISTIC phase IIIb study. Rheumatology 2012;51:2204-2214.

64. Weinblatt ME, Fleischmann R, van Vollenhoven RF et al. Twenty-eight-week results from the REALISTIC phase IIIb randomized trial: efficacy, safety and predictability of response to certolizumab pegol in a diverse rheumatoid arthritis population. Arthritis Res Ther 2015;17:325.

65. Emery P, Fleischmann RM, Moreland LW et al. Golimumab, a human anti–tumor necrosis factor alpha monoclonal antibody, injected subcutaneously everyfour weeks in methotrexate-naive patients withactive rheumatoid arthritis. Arthritis Rheum 2009;60:2272-2283.

66. Emery P, Fleischmann R, van der Heijde D et al. The effects of golimumab on radiographic progression in rheumatoid arthritis. Arthritis Rheum 2011;63:1200-1210.

67. Emery P, Fleischmann RM, Strusberg I et al. Efficacy and safety of subcutaneous golimumab in methotrexate-naïve patients with rheumatoid arthritis: 5-year results of the GO-BEFORE trial. Arthritis Care Res 2015, online Oct 15.

68. Kremer JM, Genant HK, Moreland LW et al. Effects of abatacept in patients with methotrexate-resistant active rheumatoid arthritis. Ann Intern Med 2006;144: 865-876.

69. Genant HK, Peterfy CG, Westhovens R et al. Abatacept inhibits progression of structural damage in rheumatoid arthritis: results from the longterm extension of the AIM trial. Ann Rheum Dis 2008;67:1084-1089.

70. Kremer JM, Peterfy C, RussellAS et al. Longterm safety, efficacy, and inhibition of structural damage progression over 5 years of treatment with abatacept in patients with rheumatoid arthritis in the abatacept in inadequate responders to methotrexate trial. J Rheumatol 2014;41: 1077-1087.

71. Genovese MC, Schiff M, Luggen M et al. Efficacy and safety of the selective costimulation modulator abatacept following 2 years of treatment in patients with rheumatoid arthritis and an inadequate response to anti-tumour necrosis factor therapy. Ann Rheum Dis 2008;67: 547-554.

72. Emery P, Burmester GR, Bykerk VP et al. Evaluating drugfree remission with abatacept in early rheumatoid arthritis: results from the phase 3b, multicentre, randomised, activecontrolled AVERT study of 24 months, with a 12-month, double-blind treatment period. Ann Rheum Dis 2015;74:19-26.

73. Schiff M, Weinblatt ME, Valente R et al. Head-to-head comparison of subcutaneous abatacept versus adalimumab for rheumatoid arthritis: two-year efficacy and safety findings from AMPLE trial. Ann Rheum Dis 2014; 73:86-94.

74. Emery P, Deodhar A, Rigby WF, et al. Efficacy and safety of different doses and retreatment of rituximab: a randomised, placebo-controlled trial in patients who are biological naive with active rheumatoid arthritis and an inadequate response to methotrexate (Study Evaluating Rituximab's Efficacy in MTX iNadequaterEsponders (SERENE). Ann Rheum Dis 2010;69:1629-1635.

75. Tak PP, Rigby WF, Rubbert-Roth A, et al. IMAGE Investigators. Inhibition of joint damage and improved clinical outcomes with rituximab plus methotrexate in early active rheumatoid arthritis: the IMAGE trial. Ann Rheum Dis 2011; 70:39-46.

76. Edwards JCW, Szczepanski L, Szechinski J et al. Efficacy of B-cell–targeted therapy with rituximab in patients with rheumatoid arthritis.N Engl J Med 2004;350: 2572-2581.

77. Wendler J, Burmester GR, Sörensen H et al. Rituximab in patients with rheumatoid arthritis in routine practice (GERINIS): 6-year results from a prospective, multicentre, noninterventional study in 2,484 patients. Arthritis Res Ther 2014;16:R80.

78. Richter A, Strangfeld A, Herzer P et al. Sustainability of rituximab therapy in different treatment strategies: results of a 3-year followup of a German Biologics Register. Arthritis Care Res 2014;66:1627-1633.

79. Kremer JM, Blanco R, Brzosko M, et al. Tocilizumab inhibits structural joint damage in rheumatoid arthritis patients with inadequate responses to methotrexate: results from the double-blind treatment phase of a randomized placebo-controlled trial of tocilizumab safety and prevention of structural joint damage at one year. Arthritis Rheum 2011;63:609-621.

80. Genovese MC, McKay JD, Nasonov EL, et al. Interleukin-6 receptor inhibition with tocilizumab reduces disease activity in rheumatoid arthritis with inadequate response to disease-modifying antirheumatic drugs: the tocilizumab in combination with traditional disease-modifying antirheumatic drug therapy study. Arthritis Rheum 2008;58:2968-2980

81. Smolen JS, Beaulieu A, Rubbert-Roth A, et al; OPTION Investigators. Effect of interleukin-6 receptor inhibition with tocilizumab in patients with rheumatoid arthritis (OPTION study): a double-blind, placebo-controlled, randomised trial. Lancet 2008;371:987-997.

82. Emery P, Keystone E, Tony HP, et al. IL-6 receptor inhibition with tocilizumab improves treatment outcomes in patients with rheumatoid arthritis refractory to anti-tumour necrosis factor biologicals: results from a 24-week multicentre-randomised placebo-controlled trial. Ann Rheum Dis 2008; 67:1516-1523.

83. Dougados M, Kissel K, Sheeran T, et al. Adding tocilizumab or switching to tocilizumab monotherapy in methotrexate inadequate responders: 24-week symptomatic and structural results of a 2-year randomised controlled strategy trial in rheumatoid arthritis (ACT-RAY). Ann Rheum Dis 2013;72:43-50.

84. Dougados M, Kissel K, Conaghan PG et al. Clinical, radiographic and immunogenic effects after 1 year of tocilizumab-based treatment strategies in rheumatoid arthritis: the ACT-RAY study. Ann Rheum Dis 2014;73: 803-809.

85. Burmester GR, Rubbert-Roth A, Cantagrel A, et al. A randomised, double-blind, parallel-group study of the safety and efficacy of subcutaneous tocilizumab versus intravenous tocilizumab in combination with traditional disease-modifying antirheumatic drugs in patients with moderate to severe rheumatoid arthritis (SUMMACTA study). Ann Rheum Dis 2014; 73:69-74.

86. Genovese MC, Rubbert-Roth A, Smolen JS et al. Longterm safety and efficacy of tocilizumab in patients with rheumatoid arthritis: A cumulative analysis of up to 4.6 years of exposure. J Rheumatol 2013;40:768-780.

87. Strangfeld A, Richter A, Herzer P et al. Risk for lower intestinal perforations in RA patients treated with tocilizumab in comparison to treatment with TNF inhibitors, rituximab, abatacept or conventional synthetic DMARDs. Arthritis Rheum 2015;67(Suppl.10),Abstr. 2051.

88. Huizinga TWJ, Conaghan PG, Martin-Mola E et al. Clinical and radiographic outcomes at 2 years and the effect of tocilizumab discontinuation following sustained remission in the second and third year of the ACT-RAY study. Ann Rheum Dis 2015;74:35-43.

89. Genovese MC, Fleischmann R, Kivitz AJ et al. Sarilumab plus methotrexate in patients with active rheumatoid arthritis and inadequate response to methotrexate: Results of a Phase III Study. Arthritis Rheumatol 2015; 67:1424-1437.

90. Fleischmann R, van Adelsberg J, Lin Y et al. Sarilumab and nonbiologic disease-modifying antirheumatic drugs in patients with active rheumatoid arthritis and inadequate response or intolerance to tumor necrosis factor inhibitors. Arthritis Rheumatol 2017;69:277-290.

91. Nam JL, Ramiro S, Gaujoux-Viala C et al. Efficacy of biological disease-modifying antirheumatic drugs: a systematic literature review informing the 2013 update of the EULAR recommendations for the management of rheumatoid arthritis. Ann Rheum Dis 2014;73:516-528.

92. Desai RJ, Hansen RA, Rao JK et al. Mixed treatment comparison of the treatment discontinuations of biologic disease-modifying antirheumatic drugs in adults with rheumatoid arthritis. Ann Pharmacother 2012;46: 1491-1505.

93. Fleischmann R, Mysler E, Hall S et al. Efficacy and safety of tofacitinib monotherapy, tofacitinib with methotrexate, and adalimumab with methotrexate in patients with rheumatoid arthritis (ORAL Strategy): a phase 3b/4, double-blind, head-to-head, randomised controlled trial. Lancet 2017;390:457-468.

94. Fleischmann R, Schiff M, van der Heijde D et al. Baricitinib, methotrexate, or combination in patients with rheumatoid arthritis and no or limited prior disease-modifying antirheumatic drug treatment. Arthritis Rheumatol 2017:506-517.

95. Fleischmann R, Takeuchi T, Schiff M et al. Efficacy and safety of long-term baricitinib with and without methotrexate for the treatment of rheumatoid arthritis: Experience with baricitinib monotherapy continuation or after switching from methotrexate monotherapy or baricitinib plus methotrexate. Arthritis Care Res 2020;72: 1112-1121

96. Buch M, Wells AF, Rubbert-Roth A et al. A comparative analysis of upadacitinib monotherapy and upadacitinib combination therapy for the treatment of rheumatoid arthritis from two phase 3 trial. Ann Rheum Dis 2019;78(Suppl.2):356.

97. Westhovens R, Rigby WFC, van der Heijde D et al. Filgotinib in combination with methotrexate or as monotherapy versus methotrexate monotherapy inpatients with active rheumatoid arthritis and limitedor no prior exposure to methotrexate: the phase 3, randomised controlled FINCH 3 trial. Ann Rheum Dis 3031;80:727-738.

5. Influence of methotrexate on radiographic progression

The destruction of the joints caused by the aggressive pannus is the decisive factor in the long-term disability threatening patients with rheumatoid arthritis (RA) (1).

> The extent of the joint destruction can be very well documented on X-ray images. To date, no other imaging method has been able to replace these for recording long-term changes. These changes to the joints that occur over time are also referred to as **radiographic progression**.

Regular X-rays of the hands and feet provide a representative picture of the disease progression with a close statistical correlation to the destruction of other joints (2, 3). Semi-quantitative scoring methods that record the changes in the hands and feet are a very reliable measurement of radiographic progression over long periods of time. The close association between the functional impairment described by the patient and the measured radiographic progression has been clearly demonstrated (4).

To qualify as a disease-modifying drug, it must be able to delay or stop radiographic progression. The following will show how well the disease-modifying effect of methotrexate (MTX) is documented for RA.

> The radiographic progression, which can be measured using X-ray scoring methods, correlates closely with the loss of function in patients with RA over the long term. Slowing down, standstill or even reduction in radiographic progression in the sense of tissue repair is considered evidence of the disease-modifying effect of a drug.

5.1. Radiographic progression in open long-term studies

In the 1980s, a number of studies were conducted on the efficacy of MTX in RA. None of these studies included longer placebo-controlled treatment phases.

Kremer and Lee (5) treated 29 patients with an average of 12 mg MTX for 29 months. X-rays of the hands and feet were available for only 11 patients at baseline and after 2 years. An experienced radiologist did not detect any deterioration on X-rays in any patient, but did detect a reduction in soft tissue swelling in 6 patients and a significant improvement of erosions (related to shape, appearance, size or number) in 7 patients.

The same cohort was examined after an average of 54 months and after 90 months (6). Of the remaining 18 patients, follow-up X-rays of 17 patients were evaluable after 90 months. Deterioration was seen in 9 patients, and no change was seen in 8. At this time, all X-rays had also been evaluated using the variation of the Sharp score described by Fries et al. (7). The mean erosion score (ES) had increased from 56 at baseline to 63 after 2 years, 67 after 5 years, and 72 after 8 years, with only the change after 8 years differing significantly (p=0.016) from the baseline value. The joint space narrowing score increased from 88 at baseline to 94 after 2 years, to 98 after 5 years (p=0.023), and to 106 after 8 years (p=0.007). The total score of 144 at baseline and 178 (43% of the maximum score of 412) after 8 years illustrates the severity of the disease in these patients.

In the controlled study by Weinblatt et al. (8) with 28 patients over 6 months, the patients initially received 7.5 mg MTX per week or placebo. Of these, 26 patients switched to an open-label extension phase in which all patients received MTX. The mean starting dose for MTX in the open-label extension phase was 14 mg, which was reduced to 10 mg after 12 months, to 9 mg after 24 months and to 8.6 mg per week after 36 months. 18 patients were still taking part in the study after 24 months and 16 after 36 months. X-rays of the hands of 14 patients were available at the start and after 28 months at the earliest: 6 had worsened, 3 had remained unchanged and 5 had improved in terms of the number and size of the erosions, some with healing. After 84 months (9), 6 of 10 evaluable patients showed progression in the number and size of erosions, deformities and joint space narrowing, no progression in 3 patients and healing of erosions in one case. The 4 patients without progression showed a clinical "substantial" response, defined as improvement in joint indices by >50% and in the overall assessment by physician and patient by at least 2 on a 5-point scale.

Sany et al. (10) found that in 41 patients with severe RA with an average disease duration of 13 years during an observation period of 31 months, despite clinical improvement, joint changes worsened in 84% of cases and stabilization occurred in only 6 cases (16%).

The same group later reported on the course of 29 patients with early RA and an average disease duration of 7 (2-60) months (11). X-ray images were available before starting MTX therapy and after 13±4 months. The X-ray images were evaluated using a modified Larsen score (12) and the van der Heijde Sharp score (vdH Sharp score) (13). Both scoring methods showed significant progression (in the Larsen score $p=0.001$, in the vdH Sharp score $p=0.034$). However, according to the previously established definition that a score increase below 15 points does not indicate progression, 23 (Larsen score) and 24 (vdH Sharp score) patients achieved stabilization.

In a study by Hanrahan et al. (14), 128 patients were treated with MTX. 75 patients were observed for 2 years and 49 for 3 years. X-rays were available for 47 patients at inclusion and after 2 years. 15 showed a significant deterioration, 18 showed no change, and no case clearly improved. Patients with severe radiographic deterioration were also significantly worse clinically during the 2-year period.

In another open study by Drosos et al. (15), 23 of 35 patients achieved clinical remission and 12 showed a significant improvement. X-rays of the hands before and 24 months after starting MTX treatment were assessed using a scoring method slightly modified from the Larsen method. The mean score did not increase significantly from the baseline value of 15 (±13) during treatment to 19 (±16, $p>0.5$). Stabilization of the erosions was described in 20 patients and deterioration in 15.

Overall, the open studies do not allow a reliable statement as to whether MTX influences radiographic progression or not due to

- their extremely small case numbers,
- the widely varying MTX dose and
- study designs that are not controlled over longer periods of time.

5.2. Comparison of progression before and during methotrexate treatment

The effect of treatment on radiographic progression can also be assessed, with some limitations, by comparing progression in a phase before the start of therapy with progression during the therapy.

In the study by Nordstrom et al. (16), X-ray images of the hands of 18 patients were taken an average of 33 months before starting MTX treatment and 30 months afterwards and evaluated using the Sharp score. There was a monthly increase of 0.041 Sharp score units per joint before MTX and of 0.043 Sharp score units during MTX treatment.

Reykdal et al. (17) described a reduction in the monthly progression rate in 29 months from an average of 0.58 score units before starting MTX therapy to 0.38 score units in the 33 months using MTX applying a modification of the Sharp score in 50 patients.

Wittenborg et al. (18) also found a slowing of radiographic progression in 70 patients during MTX treatment lasting an average of 28 months compared to a pre-observation period.

Rau et al. (19) compared the radiographic progression in 31 patients with clinically effective MTX treatment over 4 years with clinically ineffective pretreatment with parenteral gold over an average of 2.2 years. During MTX treatment, significantly fewer joints deteriorated from Larsen stage 0 to stage I or II than in the period before. In the case of joints in higher Larsen stages, however, there was no difference between the treatment phases. The mean progression rate of the Larsen score per joint was significantly lower ($p<0.01$) in the hands at 0.005 per month than during the previous gold treatment (0.03 per month). In the forefeet, however, there was no difference in the Larsen index between the gold and MTX phases (0.010 vs 0.011 per month per joint). During MTX treatment, the number of joints with radiographic signs of activity – soft tissue swelling, new marginal erosions, subchondral osteoporosis – decreased continuously, while the number of joints with secondary osteoarthritis, indicating local inactivation of synovitis, increased.

In summary, the studies comparing radiographic progression during MTX treatment with progression before the start of therapy provide clear indications, but for methodological reasons no firm evidence, of a slowing of radiographic progression by MTX.

5.3. Comparison of progression using methotrexate vs other basic therapeutic agents

Comparisons of two effective DMARDs can only reveal the relative difference in progression inhibition between the two substances.

5.3.1. Comparison with azathioprine

In a Canadian randomized blinded study (20), 21 patients were treated for 6 months with 15 mg MTX per week or with 150 mg azathioprine (AZA) daily. Further treatment after 24 weeks was left to the treating rheumatologists. X-rays of the hands of all patients could be assessed using the Sharp score at the start, and of 14 (9) patients from the MTX group and 16 (12) patients from the AZA group after 24 (52) weeks. There was a significant increase in both groups but no difference between the groups.

In a large comparative study with 209 patients who received increasing doses of AZA, MTX or the combination of both drugs, Willkens et al. (21) found a trend towards more progression in the AZA group compared to the MTX and combination groups, but no significant difference between the treatment groups, when analyzing 178 patients with available X-ray images at baseline and after 48 weeks using the Sharp score.

In 1991, Jeurissen et al. (22) published the radiographic results of a 48-week double-blind comparative study of MTX with AZA. After 24 and 48 weeks, there were significantly fewer new erosions (difference 2.0 [95% CI 0.2-3.9] and 3.5 [95% CI 1.3-5.8] after 24 and 48 weeks, respectively) and a significantly smaller increase in the vdH Sharp score (difference 2.8 [95% CI 0.2-5.2] and 3.9 [95% CI 0.3-7.4]). This difference continued in the second year of treatment and was still evident after 4 years, although it was no longer significant because notably more patients had switched from the AZA group to the MTX group during the follow-up phase (n=21) than vice versa (n=5).

5.3.2. Comparison with auranofin

In the 9-month comparative study between oral gold (auranofin, AF) and MTX published in 1993 by Weinblatt et al. (23), X-ray images from the start of the study and after 9 months were available for evaluation in 95 of 103 MTX patients and in 72 of 80 AF patients. With comparable baseline values, the increase in the MTX group was significantly lower in both the ES with 0.6 versus 1.7 units ($p=0.04$) and the joint space narrowing score with 0.4 versus 1.4 units ($p=0.007$) compared to the AF group.

5.3.3. Comparison with aurothiomalate

In a double-blind comparative study published by Rau et al. (24, 25) conducted bicentrically in Ratingen and Bad Abbach, 87 patients with early erosive RA received parenteral gold (50 mg aurothiomalate, ATM) or 15 mg MTX per week intramuscularly. The increase in the modified Larsen score (26) was 3.4 in the MTX group and 2.6 in the ATM group in the first 6 months, and 2.6 in the MTX group and 2.2 in the ATM group in the second 6 months. The differences between the treatment groups were not significant, but the reduction in progression in the second half of the year compared to the first half of the year was significant in both groups ($p<0.05$). The number of joints with new erosions also decreased significantly in both groups compared to the first half of the year. In a later analysis after three years of observation (27), the X-ray images were analyzed using the Ratingen score (28). The increase in the Ratingen score in the second and third year of treatment was significantly lower than in the first year, at 3.0 and 2.3 units in the MTX group and 2.1 and 2.6 units in the ATM group ($p<0.001$). The increase in the number of erosive joints also decreased significantly from 4.6 (MTX) and 3.1 (ATM) in the first year to 1.5 and 2.2 in the second year and 0.9 and 1.4 in the third year. The differences between the treatment groups were not significant.

5.3.4. Comparison with sulfasalazine

A three-arm study by Dougados et al. (29) compared the effects of sulfasalazine (SSZ) (n=68), MTX (n=69) and the combination of both drugs (n=69) in early RA (disease duration <1 year). After one year, there was a weak trend towards a lower progression of the vdH-Sharp score in the combination group (+3.5 vdH Sharp score units) compared to the monotherapy groups, which were not significantly different from each other (SSZ group +4.6; MTX group +4.5).

5.3.5. Comparison with leflunomide

In 1999, Strand et al. (30) published a study conducted only in North America with the abbreviation US301 (ULTRA study), in which leflunomide (LEF) was compared with MTX and placebo and in which X-ray images of hands and feet were taken at the beginning and after 52 weeks and assessed using the Sharp score. The radiographic progression in the LEF group (n=131) was just on the border of significance, with a score increase of 0.53 in the Total Sharp Score (TSS), and less pronounced than the increase of 0.88 in the MTX group (n=138). In both groups, the change in TSS was considerably smaller than expected when calculating a linear extrapolation of the previous progression from the TSS at inclusion divided by the disease duration: 3.3 TSS units per year in the LEF group and 3.5 TSS units per year in the MTX group). After 2 years, the increase in TSS was greater in the LEF group with 1.6 units than in the MTX group with 1.2 units, but once again not significantly different (95% CI –1.39 to 2.19, p= 0.659) (31).

The results on inhibition of radiographic progression in all approval-relevant LEF studies were summarized by Sharp et al. (32). In contrast to US301, the study conducted in Europe with significantly more subjects, abbreviated MN302, showed significantly lower progression in TSS after one year in the MTX group (n=324) at 1.6 TSS units compared to the LEF group (n=302) at 2.5 TSS units. However, this difference was not significant (p=0.3; 95% CI: –2.2 to 7.4). Nevertheless, compared to the expected progression of 6.7 in the LEF group and 6.5 in the MTX group, the measured progression in both groups was considerably lower. The percentage of patients with relevant radiographic progression (increase in erosion score >3 units) was again almost the same at 10% in the LEF group versus 11% in the MTX group (p=0.9).

5.3.6. Comparison with various other DMARDs

As early as 1992, Alarcon et al. (33) published a meta-analysis of 553 RA patients treated with MTX compared to those treated with other DMARDs, which also included data from studies that were still ongoing or only published in abstract form. In this analysis, both groups showed a similarly severe disease progression. The patients treated with MTX progressed less than those treated with AZA, but not than those treated with parenteral gold.

> The data from the comparative studies with other conventional DMARDs provide strong arguments for the assumption that MTX slows down the radiographic progression in RA. However, evidence of superiority over other conventional DMARDs could only be found for the comparison with AF.

5.4. Comparison of methotrexate / placebo with respect to inhibition of progression

There are only very few studies that compare radiographic progression under MTX with a placebo group. The best data stem from the ULTRA study already cited, in which LEF was compared with MTX and placebo (26). In the MTX group, the increase in TSS was significantly lower at 0.9 units than in the placebo group (2.2 units, p=0.02). In the last Cochrane analysis on the effectivity of MTX, only the data from this study were included regarding the effect of MTX on radiographic progression (34) and they were interpreted in such a way that, beyond the effect in the placebo group, 8% of patients treated with MTX for over a year can achieve a relevant reduction in radiographic progression of at least three Sharp Score units.

The second placebo-controlled study with MTX by van Dongen et al. (35) was not conducted in a cohort of patients with confirmed RA. Rather, it included only patients with early undifferentiated arthritis who did not yet meet the then valid 1987 classification criteria for the diagnosis of RA (36) at the time of inclusion in the study. Of the 55 patients in each treatment group, 22 in the MTX group and 29 in the placebo group met the diagnostic criteria for RA over a period of up to 30 months. X-rays of 51 patients from each group were evaluable at baseline and after 18 months. Significantly fewer patients in the MTX group (6 vs 14, p=0.046) showed an increase in the vdH Sharp score that was greater than the smallest measurable difference. In patients with erosive changes, the individual progression in the MTX group was also significantly lower than in the placebo group (p=0.035). In patients with detected CCP antibodies, progression was also significantly lower (p=0.03). Even though the patients in this study did not have diagnosed RA at the time of inclusion, radiographic progression was significantly reduced, especially in those patients who developed RA during the course of the study (☞ Figure 5.1).

The placebo-controlled studies prove that MTX reduces radiographic progression, even if this statement is based on very limited data. For ethical reasons, longer, placebo-controlled studies in RA, which could provide a broader basis for this data, are no longer being carried out.

5.5. Comparison of methotrexate / biologics or small molecules (JAK inhibitors) with respect to inhibition of progression

Approval studies for new substances for the treatment of RA, including biologics, were mainly carried out on patients who had a high level of disease activity despite treatment with MTX. These so-called MTX non-responder studies cannot help clarify whether and to what extent MTX inhibits radiographic progression.

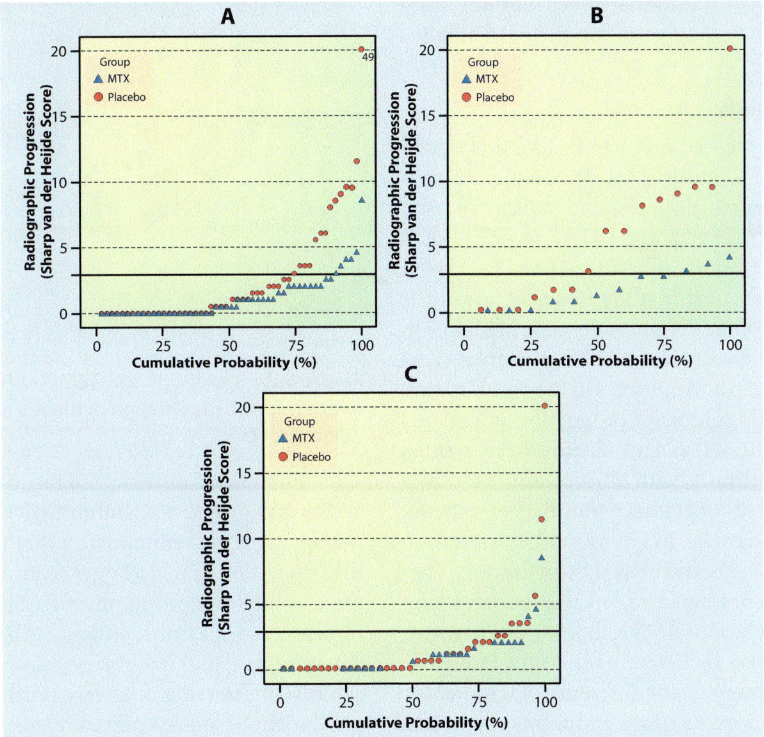

Figure 5.1: Effectivity of MTX treatment in patients with early undifferentiated arthritis (= with probable RA) according to van Dongen et al. (35). The possible radiographic progression (Sharp vdH score) was calculated over 18 months in 102 patients. The horizontal lines correspond to the smallest measurable difference.
A: Total group (n=102, p=0.15). **B**: Group of anti-CCP antibody-positive patients (n=27, p=0.03). **C**: Group of anti-CCP antibody-negative patients (n=75, p=0.46).
The three p-values are based on the comparison of MTX vs placebo. Explanation of the results see text.

Because it must be assumed that structural damage to the joints, once it has occurred, is only rarely and then only partially reversible, a longer placebo-controlled phase in clinical studies for RA is no longer ethically justifiable. For this reason, at least since the beginning of the biologics era, studies for early RA have been designed in such a way that MTX-naive patients are switched to MTX or the comparative therapy. However, this study design can only make a statement about the relative potency of the drugs for inhibiting radiographic progression. The use of the concept of calculating the expected radiographic progression from the duration of the disease and the damage already present at the time of inclusion in the study is all the more problematic the shorter the duration of the disease and is therefore not an option for these patient groups. Only studies that include a combination treatment arm in addition to the two therapies being tested as monotherapy can provide information on the additional effect that MTX has on radiographic progression compared to biologic monotherapy.

TEMPO study

The first study to be conducted using this design was the TEMPO study (37). Patients were randomly assigned to double-blind treatment with MTX (n=228), etanercept (ETA) (n=223) or a combination of both substances (n=231). What was unusual about this study was that, given the long duration of the disease at the time of inclusion in the study (6.8 years in the MTX group, 6.3 years in the ETA group and 6.8 years in the combination group), a not insignificant proportion of patients (42%, 42% and 44%) had already been treated with MTX previously, with MTX treatment having been interrupted for at least 6 months beforehand. This means that the MTX monotherapy group could have been disadvantaged from the outset because it could not be ruled out that patients who had previously stopped MTX therapy due to insufficient effect were included in the study. However, no statistically significant difference was found for any of the important study endpoints, including radiographic progression, when comparing patients who had previously received MTX with those who had not received MTX. The MTX group was significantly inferior to the other two groups in the previously defined primary endpoint, the numerical ACR response, measured over time as the area under the curve (ACR-N AUC), but in all other clinical endpoints only the combination group was significantly better than each of the monotherapy groups. Complete sets of X-ray images from 212 (MTX), 212 (ETA) and 218 (combination) patients were available for the radiographic evaluation after 52 weeks. Despite the largely identical clinical efficacy of the monotherapy groups, the vdH-Sharp score in the MTX group increased significantly (p=0.0469) by 2.8 units compared to only 0.52 in the ETA group, but was clearly significant compared to the negative score of -0.54 in the combination group (p<0.0001; ☞ Figure 5.2). The combination group was also significantly better than the ETA group (p=0.0006).

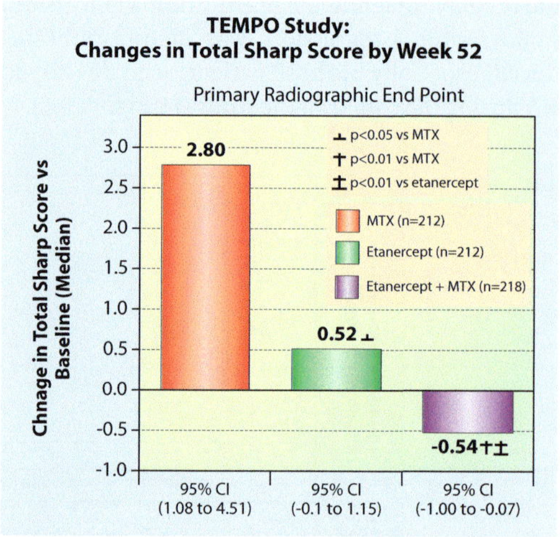

Figure 5.2: Results of the TEMPO study. **CI**: Confidence interval. Explanation of the results see text. Modified after (37).

This difference can therefore be attributed to the additional progression-inhibiting effect of MTX therapy. It is also noteworthy that this study was the first to find that in a larger treatment group, i.e. the combination group, the vdH Sharp score was negative at –0.5 units, which, with a 95% confidence interval that was also negative (–1.0 to –0.1), can be considered a relatively reliable sign of improvement or at least partial repair. This observation that the progression was significantly greater in the MTX group than in the other two groups and that the combination group showed significantly less progression than the other two treatment groups, and even a negative progression of –0.8 and –0.1 compared to the initial findings, was also confirmed in the continuation of the study after two (38) and three (39) years.

CAMEO study

In a Canadian phase IV study (40), 256 patients with active RA despite treatment with MTX were randomized after 6 months of additional treatment with ETA to continue treatment with either the combination of MTX and ETA (n=107) or with ETA as monotherapy (n=98). After 24 months, the mean vdH-modified total sharp score (mTSS) had increased by 0.4 units in the group in which MTX had been discontinued, while no increase was found in the group that continued to receive MTX. Whether this difference was significant was not calculated. However, this study supports the assumption of a (small) additional effect of MTX therapy on radiographic progression.

PREMIER study

In the PREMIER study (41), in which patients with early erosive or seropositive RA received either adalimumab (ADA) (n=274, 94% erosive at inclusion) or MTX (n=257, 95% erosive) or the combination of both drugs (n=268, 93% erosive), the increase in TSS after 6, 12 and 24 months was significantly (p<0.001) greater in the MTX group with 3.5, 5.7 and 10.4 units, respectively, than in the ADA group with 2.1, 3.0 and 5.5 units and in the combination group with 0.8, 1.3 and 1.9 units, respectively (☞ Figure 5.3).

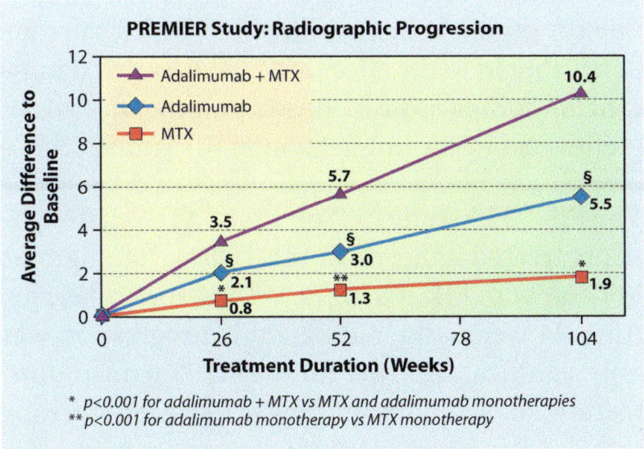

Figure 5.3: PREMIER study: increase in the Total Sharp Score 26, 52 and 104 weeks after the start of the study. Modified according to (40).

The differences between the combination group and the ADA group were also always significant (p<0.001 after 6 and 24 months, p=0.002 after 12 months). In this study, MTX in combination with ADA clearly increased the inhibition of radiographic progression compared to ADA monotherapy.

GO-BEFORE study

A similar study design was also used in the study with golimumab (GLM) in MTX-naive RA, the GO-BEFORE study (42). 160 patients were treated with MTX (group 1) and 159 patients each with GLM 100 mg (group 2) or with the combination of MTX with 50 mg GLM (group 3) or with 100 mg GLM (group 4). In group 1, the increase in the vdH Sharp score after 28 and 52 weeks was 1.1 and 1.4 units – significantly lower than in the MTX group of the PREMIER study. In group 2, an increase by 0.7 and 1.3 units was found, in group 3 by 0.7 and 0.7 and in group 4 by 0.01 and 0.07 units. The increase was only significantly lower in group 4 at both time points and in group 3 after 52 weeks compared to the MTX group. Even though the radiographic progression in group 4 was almost zero and in group 2 almost as high as in group 1, one can assume that this considerable difference between group 2 and group 4, which only differed in the additional administration of MTX, was also significant; unfortunately, this information is not available in the publication.

ACT-RAY study

Another study design, which also allows a statement to be made about a possible influence of MTX on radiographic progression in combination with a biologic, was implemented in the ACT-RAY study, in which patients who had previously responded inadequately to MTX were treated either with tocilizumab (TCZ) alone (n=276) or with the combination of TCZ with MTX (n=277). After 24 weeks, the increase in the group that continued with combination therapy with MTX in the Genant-modified Total Sharp Score (GSS) (43) was 0.08 units and in the ES was -0.01 units, but not significantly reduced compared to the group that continued treatment with TCZ alone, in which the increase in the GSS was 0.22 (p=0.26) and in the ES was 0.11 (p=0.066) units (44). After 52 weeks, the difference in the GSS was still not significant at 0.18 versus 0.35 (p=0.36), but the difference in the ES was clearly significant at 0.03 versus 0.15 (p=0.001) (45). After 104 weeks, however, the overall very small difference was significant both in the GSS at 0.35 versus 0.95 (p=0.035) and in the ES at –0.03 versus 0.26 (p=0.037) (46).

Registry data and non-interventional studies

Additional findings revealing a possible additive effect of MTX on radiographic progression in combination with biologics could also be drawn from the analyses of registry data or from non-interventional studies in which radiographic progression was recorded and compared in the combination group vs the biologics monotherapy group. These studies had the great advantage that, without strict inclusion and exclusion criteria, they were much closer to the treatment reality (real world evidence) than the results from randomized clinical studies. However, such analyses including examination of radiographic progression have so far only been published in the Danish Biologics Registry (DANBIO) and in the large non-interventional PRERA study with ETA conducted in Germany.

In the analysis of 930 patients from the DANBIO registry (47), no significant difference in radiographic progression was found between patients treated with the TNF inhibitors ADA, ETA and infliximab (INX) as monotherapy and those treated in combination with MTX. In this retrograde analysis, however, an influence of the result based on the indication in the sense of "confounding by indication" could not be ruled out, because it can be assumed that MTX was more likely to be retained as a combination partner if there was a higher disease activity or a more severe course of the disease.

The same limitation also applies to the results of the PRERA study (48), in which radiographic progression was measured in 511 patients with RA and 167 patients with PsA after starting treatment with ETA. No difference in radiographic progression was found between patients treated with ETA alone and those who also received MTX.

The lack of evidence of an additional progression-inhibiting effect of combination treatment with MTX could therefore best be explained by indication bias in these studies.

Studies with JANUS kinase inhibitors (small molecules)

In the approval studies for the JAK inhibitors baricitinib (BAR) and filgotinib (FIL), studies were also carried out in MTX-naive patients, comparing either MTX or the respective JAK inhibitor or the combination of the JAK inhibitor with MTX.

In contrast, in the development program for tofacitinib (TFB) and upadacitinib (UPA) in MTX-naive patients, only the respective monotherapy groups were compared with each other, without including a combination group. In the ORAL-START study with TFB (49), it was shown that the radiographic progression was significantly lower in the two TFB groups (5 or 10 mg daily) compared to the MTX group. The same result was also found in the SELECT-Early study with UPA (15 or 30 mg daily) (50). There was no combination group in either study. Therefore, these studies do not allow any conclusions to be drawn about an additional effect of MTX in combination with TFB.

In the RA BEGIN study with BAR (51), the radiographic progression measured with the mTSS after 24 and 52 weeks was only significantly lower in the combination group than in the MTX group with 0.29 and 0.40 mTSS units, and with 0.26 and 0.34 units in the erosion score (ES) (mTSS 0.61 and 1.02 mTSS units and 0.47 and 0.81 ES units, respectively). In the BAR monotherapy group, the increases of 0.39 and 0.81 units in the mTSS and of 0.33 and 0.55 units in the ES were not significantly lower than in the MTX group. The proportion of patients without measurable radiographic progression (defined as a change in the mTSS of <0.5 or even of 0.0) was also only significantly higher in the combination group than in the MTX monotherapy group. The radiographic progression was therefore lower in the combination group vs the BAR monotherapy group. Whether this effect, which can only be attributed to the effect of MTX, was also significant in comparison to BAR monotherapy is not mentioned in the publication of the study.

The FINCH 3 study (52) observed MTX-naive patients treated either with FIL 100 or 200 mg plus MTX or with FIL 200 mg or MTX as monotherapy. After 24 weeks, the radiographic progression was only significantly lower for the FIL 200 mg monotherapy dose than in the MTX monotherapy group. After 52 weeks, the progression in all other groups was significantly lower than in the TX monotherapy group. However, the difference between the FIL 200 mg monotherapy group and the 200 mg MTX combination group was minimal at 0.23 vs 0.21 mTSS units, which was confirmed in the post hoc analysis (53) of the subgroup of patients with 4 unfavorable prognostic factors (mTSS

0.41 in the combination group vs 0.40 in the FIL monotherapy group).

In summary, the studies cited suggest that pertaining the treatment with biologics, particularly TNF blockers, to a much lesser extent also TCZ and questionably also the JAK inhibitor BAR, an additional effect on radiographic progression can be achieved with the combined administration of MTX. Such an effect has not been demonstrated for FIL and has not been investigated for TFB and UPA. In the case of biologics, it is not possible to define with certainty how much of this effct is directly attributable to the progression-inhibiting effect of MTX in the sense of an additive effect to the biologic, or whether it is an indirect consequence of the inhibition of antibody formation against the biologic, which then allows the biologic to work more effectively.

5.6. References

1. Scott DL, Pugner K, Kaarela K, et al. The links between joint damage and disability in rheumatoid arthritis. Rheumatology 2000;39:122-32.

2. Scott DL, Coulton BL, Popert AJ. Long term progression of joint damage in rheumatoid arthritis. Ann Rheum Dis 1986;45:373-8.

3. Kuper HH, van Leeuwen MA, van Riel PL, Prevoo ML, Houtman PM, Lolkema WF, et al. Radiographic damage in large joints in early rheumatoid arthritis: relationship with radiographic damage in hands and feet, disease activity, and physical disability. Br J Rheumatol 1997; 36: 855-60.

4. Smolen JS, Aletaha D,Grisar JC, Stamm TA, Sharp JT. Estimation of a numerical value for joint damage-related physical disability in rheumatoid arthritis clinical trials. Ann Rheum Dis 2010; 69: 1058-1064.

5. Kremer JM, Lee JK. The safety and efficacy of the use of methotrexate in long-term therapy for rheumatoid arthritis. Arthritis Rheum 1986; 29: 822-31.

6. Kremer JM, Phelps CT. Long-term prospective study of the use of methotrexate in the treatment of rheumatoid arthritis. Arthritis Rheum 1992; 35: 138-145.

7. Fries JF, Bloch DA, Sharp JT, McShane DJ, Spitz P, Bluhm GB, Forrester D, Genant H, Gofton P, Richman S, Weissman B, Wolfe F: Assessment of radiologic progression in rheumatoid arthritis. a randomized, controlled trial. Arthritis Rheum 1986; 29: 1-9.

8. Weinblatt ME, Coblyn JS, Fox DA, Holdsworth DE, Glass DN, Trentham DE: Efficacy of low-dose methotrexate in rheumatoid arthritis. N Engl J Med 1985; 312: 818-822.

9. Weinblatt ME, Weissman BN, Holdsworth DE, Fraser PA, Maier AL, et al. Long-term prospective study of methotrexate in the treatment of rheumatoid arthritis. 84-month update. Arthritis Rheum 1992; 35: 129-37.

10. Sany J, Kaliski S, Couret M, et a. Radiologic progression during intramuscular methotrexate treatment of rheumatoid arthritis. J Rheumatol 1990; 17: 1636-41.

11. Maravic M, Bologna C, Daures JP, Jorgensen C, Combe B, Sany J. Radiologic progression in early rheumatoid arthritis treated with methotrexate. J Rheumatol 1999;26:262-7.

12. Larsen A. How to apply Larsen score in evaluating radiographs of rheumatoid arthritis in longterm studies. J Rheumatol 1995;22:1974-5.

13. Van der Heijde D. How to read radiographs according to the Sharp/van der Heijde method. J Rheumatol 1999;26:743-5.

14. Hanrahan PS, Scrivens GA, Russell AS. Prospective long term follow-up of methotrexate therapy in rheumatoid arthritis: Toxicity, efficacy and radiological progression. Brit J Rheum 1989; 28: 147-53.

15. Drosos AA, Karantanas AH, Psychos D, Tsampoulas C, Moutsopulos HM: Can treatment with methotrexate influence the radiological progression of rheumatoid arthritis? Clin Rheumatol 1990; 9: 342-5.

16. Nordstrom DM, West SG, Andersen PA, Sharp JT. Pulse methotrexate therapy in rheumatoid arthritis. A controlled prospective roentgenographic study. Ann Intern Med 1987; 107:797-801

17. Reykdal S, Steinsson K, Sigurjonsson K, Brekkan A. Methotrexate treatment of rheumatoid arthritis: effects on radiological progression. Scand J Rheumatology 1989; 18:221-6.

18. Wittenborg A, Ball P, Beyer HC. Radiologische Progression unter Methotrexat-Langzeittherapie (abstract). Z Rheumatol 1992; 51,(suppl2):57.

19. Rau R, Herborn G, Karger T, Werdier D. Retardation of radiologic progression in rheumatoid arthritis with methotrexate therapy. Arthritis Rheum 1991; 10: 1236-44.

20. Hamdy H, McKendry RJR, Mierins E, Liver JA: Low-dose methotrexate compared with azathioprine in the treatment of rheumatoid arthritis. Arthritis Rheum 1987; 30: 361-8.

21. Willkens RF, Sharp JT, Stablein DM, Marks CR, Wortman R. Comparison of azathioprine, methotrexate, and the combination of both in the treatment of rheumatoid arthritis. A 48 week controlled clinical trial with radiologic outcome assessment. Arthritis Rheum 1995; 38: 1799-1806.

22. Jeurissen MEC, Boerbooms AMT, van de Putte LBA, Doesburg WH and Lemmens AM. Influence of Methotrexate and Azathioprine on Radiologic Progression in Rheumatoid Arthritis: A Randomized, Double-Blind Study. Ann Intern Med. 1991;114:999-1004.

23. Weinblatt ME, Polisson R, Blotner SD, Sosman JL, Aliabadi P, Baker N, et al. The effects of drug therapy on radiographic progression of rheumatoid arthritis: results of a 36-week randomized trial comparing methotrexate and auranofin. Arthritis Rheum 1993;36:613-9.

24. Rau R, Herborn G, Menninger H, Blechschmidt J: Comparison of intramuscular methotrexate and gold sodium thiomalate in the treatment of early erosive rheumatoid arthritis: 12 month data of a double-blind parallel study of 174 patients. Brit J Rheum 1997; 36: 345-52.

25. Rau R, Herborn G, Menninger H, Sangha O. Progression in early erosive rheumatoid arthritis: 12 month results from a randomised controlled trial comparing methotrexate and gold sodium thiomalate. Brit J Rheumatol 1998; 37: 1220-6.

26. Rau R, Herborn G. A modified version of Larsen's scoring method to assess radiologic changes in rheumatoid arthritis. J Rheumatol 1995;22:1976-82

27. Rau R, Herborn G, Menninger H, Sangha O: Radiographic outcome after three years of patients with early erosive rheumatoid arthritis treated with intramuscular methotrexate or parenteral gold. Extension of a one-year double-blind study in 174 patients. Rheumatology 2002: 41: 196-204.

28. Rau R, Wassenberg S, Herborn G, Stucki G, Gebler A. A new method of scoring radiographic change in rheumatoid arthritis. J Rheumatol 1998;25:2094-106.

29. Dougados M, Combe B, Cantagrel A et al. Combination therapy in early rheumatoid arthritis: a randomised, controlled, double blind 52 week clinical trial of sulphasalazine and methotrexate compared with the single components. Ann Rheum Dis 1999; 58:220-225.

30. Strand V, Cohen S, Schiff M, Weaver A, Fleischmann R, Cannon G, Fox R, Moreland L, Olsen N, Furst D, Caldwell J, Kaine J, Sharp J, Hurley F and Löw-Friedrich I for the Leflunomide Rheumatoid Arthritis Investigators Group. Treatment of active rheumatoid arthritis with leflunomide compared with placebo and methotrexate. Arch Intern Med 1999;159: 2542-50.

31. Cohen S, Cannon GW, Schiff M, Weaver A, Fox R, Olsen N, Furst D, Sharp J, Moreland L, Caldwell J, Kaine J (for the Utilization of Leflunomide in the Treatment of Rheumatoid Arthritis Trial Investigator Group) and Strand V. Two-year, blinded, randomized, controlled trial of treatment of active rheumatoid arthritis with leflunomide compared with methotrexate. Arthritis Rheum 2001;44:1984-92.

32. Sharp JT, Strand V, Leung H, Hurley F, Loew-Friedrich I on behalf of the Leflunomide Rheumatoid Arthritis Investigators Group. Treatment with leflunomide slows radiographic progression of rheumatoid arthritis – Results from three randomized controlled trials of leflunomide in patients with active rheumatoid arthritis. Arthritis Rheum 2000;43:495-505.

33. Alarcon GS, Lopez-Mendez A, Walter J, et al. Radiographic evidence of disease progression in methotrexate-treated and nonmethotrexate disease modifying antirheumatic drug treated rheumatoid arthritis patients. A meta-analysis. J Rheumatol 1992; 19: 1868-73.

34. Lopez-Olivo MA, Siddhanamatha HR, Shea B, Tugwell P, Wells GA, Suarez-Almazor ME. Methotrexate for treating rheumatoid arthritis. Cochrane Database of Systematic Reviews 2014, Issue 6.

35. van Dongen H, van Aken J, Lard LR, Visser K, Ronday HK, Hulsmans HMJ, Speyer I, Westedt ML, Peeters AJ, Allaart CF, Toes REM, Breedveld FC, Huizinga TWJ. Efficacy of methotrexate treatment in patients with probable rheumatoid arthritis: A double-blind, randomized, placebo-controlled trial. Arthritis Rheum 2007,56:1424-1432.

36. Arnett FC, Edworthy SM, Bloch DA, McShane DJ, Fries JF, Cooper NS, et al. The American Rheumatism Association 1987 revised criteria for the classification of rheumatoid arthritis. Arthritis Rheum 1988;31:315-24.

37. Klareskog L, van der Heijde D, de Jager JP, Gough A, Kalden J, Malaise M, et al. Therapeutic effect of the combination of etanercept and methotrexate compared with each treatment alone in patients with rheumatoid arthritis: double-blind randomized controlled trial. Lancet 2004;363:675-81.

38. van der Heijde D, Klareskog L, Rodriguez-Valverde V, Codreanu C, Bolosiu H, Melo-Gomes J, Tornero-Molina J, Wajdula J, Pedersen R, Fatenejad S and TEMPO Study Investigators. Comparison of etanercept and methotrexate, alone and combined, in the treatment of rheumatoid arthritis: Two-year clinical and radiographic results from the TEMPO study, a double-blind, randomized trial. Arthritis Rheum 2006;54: 1063-1074.

39. van der Heijde D, Klareskog L, Landewé R, Bruyn GAW, Cantagrel A, Durez P, Herrero-Beaumont G, Molad Y, Codreanu C, Valentini G, Zahora R, Pedersen R, MacPeek D, Wajdula J, Fatenejad S. Disease remission and sustained halting of radiographic progression with combination etanercept and methotrexate in patients with rheumatoid arthritis. Arthritis Rheum 2007;56: 3928-3939.

40. Keystone EC, Pope JE, Thorne JC, et al. Two-year radiographic and clinical outcomes from the Canadian Methotrexate and Etanercept Outcome study in patients with rheumatoid arthritis. Rheumatology (Oxford). 2016;55:327-34.

41. Breedveld FC, Weisman MH, Kavanaugh AF, Cohen SB, Pavelka K, van Vollenhoven R, et al, for the PREMIER Investigators. The PREMIER study: a multicenter, randomized, double-blind clinical trial of combination therapy with adalimumab plus methotrexate versus methotrexate alone or adalimumab alone in patients with early, aggressive rheumatoid arthritis who had not had previous methotrexate treatment. Arthritis Rheum 2006;54:26-37.

42. Emery P, Fleischmann R, van der Heijde D, Keystone EC, Genovese MC, et al. The effects of golimumab on radiographic progression in rheumatoid arthritis: Results of randomized controlled studies on Golimimab before methotrexate therapy and golimumab after methotrexate therapy. Arthritis Rheum 2011;63:1200-1210.

43. Genant HK, Jiang Y, Peterfy C, Lu Y, Redei J, Countryman PJ. Assessment of rheumatoid arthritis using a modified scoring method on digitized and original radiographs. Arthritis Rheum 1998;41:1583-90.

44. Dougados M, Kissel K, Sheeran T, et al. Adding tocilizumab or switching to tocilizumab monotherapy in methotrexate inadequate responders: 24-week symptomatic and structural results of a 2-year randomised controlled strategy trial in rheumatoid arthritis (ACT-RAY). Ann Rheum Dis 2013;72:43-50.

45. Dougados M, Kissel K, Conaghan PG, et al. Clinical, radiographic and immunogenic effects after 1 year of tocilizumab-based treatment strategies in rheumatoid arthritis: the ACT-RAY study. Ann Rheumatic Dis 2014; 73:803-809.

46. Huizinga TWJ, Conaghan PG, Martin-Mola E, et al. Clinical and radiographic outcomes at 2 years and the effect of tocilizumab discontinuation following sustained remission in the second and third year of the ACT-RAY study. Ann Rheum Dis 2015;74:35-43.

47. Ørnbjerg LM, Østergaard M, Bøyesen P, et al. Which factors influence radiographic progression during treatment with tumor necrosis factor inhibitors in clinical practice? Re-

sults from 930 patients with rheumatoid arthritis in the nationwide Danish DANBIO registry. J Rheumatol 2014;41: 2352-60.

48. Wassenberg S, Rau R, Klopsch T, et al. Etanercept is effective and halts radiographic progression in rheumatoid arthritis and psoriatic arthritis: Final results from a German non-interventional study (PRERA). Rheumatol Ther (2022). https://doi.org/10.1007/s40744-022-00491 -4

49. Lee,EB., Fleischmann R, Hall, S et al. Tofacitinib versus methotrexate in rheumatoid arthritis. N Engl J Med 2014; 370:2377-2386

50. Peterfy CG, Strand V, Friedman A et al. Inhibition of structural joint damage progression with upadacitinib in rheumatoid arthritis: 1-year outcomes from the SELECT phase 3 program. Rheumatology (Oxford) 2022;61: 3246-3256.

52. Fleischmann R, Schiff M, van der Heijde et al. Baricitinib, methotrexate, or combination in patients with rheumatoid arthritis and no or limited prior disease-modifying antirheumatic drug treatment. Arthritis Rheumatol 2017;69:506-517.

53. Westhovens R, Rigby WFC, van der Heijde D, et al. Filgotinib in combination with methotrexate or as monotherapy versus methotrexate monotherapy in patients with active rheumatoid arthritis and limited or no prior exposure to methotrexate: the phase 3, randomised controlled FINCH 3 trial. Annals of the Rheumatic Diseases 2021;80:727-738.

54. Aletaha D, Westhovens R, Gaujoux-Viala C. Efficacy and safety of filgotinib in methotrexate-naive patients with rheumatoid arthritis with poor prognostic factors: post hoc analysis of FINCH 3. RMD Open 2021;7: e001621.

6. Methotrexate for spondyloarthritis, vasculitis and connective tissue diseases

In the treatment of rheumatoid arthritis (RA), methotrexate (MTX) is the undisputed first choice, but has also proven effective in a variety of other rheumatic diseases.

> Fortunately, the effective dose of 15 to 25 (rarely 30) mg weekly, the contraindications and adverse effects are the same for all these diseases. None of the disease entities is associated with a special risk when MTX is used.

This chapter can therefore concentrate mainly on data on the effectivity of MTX in various disease groups. For reasons of space, the studies of the highest available evidence level are discussed first and foremost.

> Of the diseases discussed in this chapter, in Germany MTX is still only approved for psoriatic arthritis (PsA).

6.1. Spondyloarthritis

As an 'exception to the rule', MTX is ineffective for ankylosing spondylitis and other forms of axial spondyloarthritis and is therefore not used in combination with TNF blockers (1). Peripheral manifestations of spondyloarthritides, on the other hand, were the first area of application of MTX in rheumatology.

6.1.1. Psoriatic arthritis

> MTX is approved for standard therapy of PsA and is clearly recommended for this purpose (2, 3).

Patients with PsA have been successfully treated with MTX for decades. The latest version of the EULAR recommendations from 2023 also recommends MTX as the first treatment of choice for patients with polyarthritis or oligoarthritis and risk factors for structural damage, especially when skin involvement is relevant (2). However, the data is nowhere near as good as for RA. In fact, successful double-blind controlled clinical trials that meet today's standards are completely lacking. In addition to numerous open studies and registry analyses, there are a total of five randomized studies: O'Brien 1962, Black 1964, Wilkens 1984, Scarpa 2008 and Kingsley 2012 (3). While the first two studies found significant differences with MTX doses that are, from today's perspective, significantly too high (up to 3 mg/kg), Wilkens' study (with 7.5-15 mg per week) only showed significant differences for the improvement in the global assessment and the extent of the skin affected by psoriasis. A trend towards joint improvement was documented, but unfortunately, in any trial, a "trend" is only an observation and does not constitute proof that a drug is actually better than the comparison substance.

Of the two randomized studies published since 2000, Scarpa et al. (4) showed advantages of MTX administration over the full six months compared to low-dose MTX administration that only began after three months (10 mg per week intramuscularly). After three months, the number of swollen and tender joints was also significantly different (4). The most recent six-month study with the mean dose of 15 mg MTX weekly (5), however, found no significant differences for the primary endpoints and was controversially discussed. It will therefore be presented in a little more detail: Of 462 patients screened, only 109 were randomized to MTX and 112 to placebo, which, however, corresponded to the sample size estimate. 21 and 23 patients, respectively, were lost to follow-up. Although numerically about twice as good, none of the three endpoints was significantly different:

- PsARC OR 1.77 (0.97-3.23), p=0.06
- ACR20 OR 2.0 (0.65-6.22), p=0.23
- DAS28 OR 1.70 (0.90-3.17), p=0.10

However, both the patients and the investigators saw an improvement with MTX (from 50 to 32 or from 41 to 23 mm on the 100 mm visual analogue scale), but not with placebo (from 50 to 42 or from 44 to 33 mm), which in each case resulted in significant differences (p=0.02 or p=0.01). Ultimately, the dose and design were certainly problematic, but the trial does not speak against the effectivity of MTX in PsA.

A Cochrane review also concludes that MTX is effective in PsA (6). In addition, there are the positive results of the (admittedly unblinded) tight-control TICOPA study (7). Overall, there is therefore little doubt about the effectivity of higher MTX doses in PsA, although the data is still not satisfactory. One difficulty is the obvious effect on skin involvement, which complicates clear, isolated conclusions about arthritis.

New data show that, in contrast to RA, there is no additional therapeutic effect of MTX in combination with TNF blockers (8-10). However, in the study by Mease et al., the MTX monotherapy arm was also apparently effective (10).

6.2. Arteritis and vasculitis

6.2.1. Giant cell arteritis

The approval of the interleukin-6 receptor blocker tocilizumab (TCZ) has significantly changed the framework for the treatment of giant cell arteritis. In the EULAR recommendations (11), MTX is still named as an alternative to TCZ. However, MTX is significantly less effective than TCZ and is now only considered clinically in exceptional cases. Nevertheless, MTX is generally effective, as shown in the meta-analysis published in 2007 by Mahr et al. (12). This analysis included all three placebo-controlled studies (Spiera 2001, Jover 2001 and Hoffman 2003) with a total of 161 patients. Individual, anonymized patient data was made available from all three studies. Although two of the three studies were negative, the meta-analysis came to a clearly positive result. For the first relapse, the RR was reduced to 0.65 using MTX with a 95% CI of 0.44 to 0.98, and for the second relapse, the RR was 0.49 (CI 0.27-0.89). Patients <75 years of age in particular benefited from MTX (RR 0.46 (CI 0.26-0.82) and 0.34 (CI 0.15-0.78)).

Interestingly, Yates et al. (13) evaluated the same three studies differently in the MTX part of their overall negative meta-analysis, namely with a non-significant RR of 0.85 (CI 0.66-1.10). However, unlike Mahr et al.'s paper, this meta-analysis was not based on individual data and therefore loses a lot of its significance.

> Although the meta-analysis of individual patient data by Mahr et al. showed the effectivity of MTX in giant cell arteritis, the significantly more effective TCZ has largely replaced this therapeutic approach.

6.2.2. Vasculitis of small and medium-sized vessels

Randomized controlled MTX studies are available for both the induction therapy of ANCA-associated vasculitides and their maintenance therapy (14). The EULAR recommendations also include MTX as an alternative for induction therapy in non-life-threatening forms and for maintenance therapy (15).

In the induction phase of the NORAM study (16), MTX (20-25 mg per week) was tested against oral cyclophosphamide (CP) in 89 patients with granulomatosis with polyangiitis (Wegener) (GPA) and 6 patients with microscopic polyangiitis (MPA), each without kidney involvement. Within 6 months, 44 of 49 MTX-treated patients (90%) and 43 of 46 CP-treated patients (94%) achieved remission, so that non-inferiority could be demonstrated (15% difference significantly rejected with p=0.041). However, MTX patients with very extensive disease (Disease Extent Index [DEI] >10) or lung involvement responded more slowly. In the follow-up (median 6 [0.1-10.8 years]), however, more patients from the MTX arm suffered a relapse after discontinuing medication after one year (17). In addition, there were no significant differences in severe and life-threatening adverse effects (with regard to the development of tumors, this was certainly still too short a follow-up). Nevertheless, MTX is a valid option as induction therapy for localized GPA and preserved renal function if followed by adequate maintenance therapy.

Rituximab is now the standard recommendation for maintenance therapy after achieving remission, because it is clearly more effective than azathioprine (AZA). AZA and MTX are considered equivalent alternatives. In the WEGENT study (18), MTX (titrated to 25 mg per week) for maintenance therapy over one year was also unable to show that it was less toxic overall than AZA (2 mg/kg body weight daily). This study included 96 patients with GPA and 30 patients with MPA.

Severe adverse events occurred in 11/63 MTX patients (18%), but only 5/63 AZA patients (8%). Events that led to treatment discontinuation were distributed 11 (17%) to 7 (11%), with only one death in the MTX arm. After two years, 75% of the patients in the MTX arm were relapse-free and alive, compared to 72% in the AZA arm. 32/44 relapses (73%) occurred after treatment was terminated. In combination with the CYCAZAREM study (19), which showed a successful switch to AZA after remission was achieved, MTX can be considered safe in maintenance therapy, but not better or with fewer side effects than AZA therapy. In any case, maintenance therapy over several years should be the goal, with at least 15 mg per week being required for MTX to be effective (20).

6.3. Connective tissue diseases

6.3.1. Systemic lupus erythematosus

MTX is recommended by EULAR for the treatment of non-renal SLE (21). Compared to other substances, the data for MTX in SLE therapy is relatively good (22). Clear evidence can be found in particular for the response to general disease activity and lupus arthritis, but also certain skin manifestations (SCLE, DLE), while the data for vasculitis, serositis and blood count changes is somewhat more limited (23). Although there is evidence of effectivity for lupus nephritis and severe CNS manifestations (intrathecal), MTX is practically not used in these indications.

In the largest controlled study to date, Fortin et al. (24) randomized 86 SLE patients to up to 20 mg MTX per week (increased from 7.5 mg in 2.5 mg increments) or placebo. More than 90% of the patients suffered from musculoskeletal involvement. Because hydroxychloroquine (HCQ) was unevenly distributed, this had to be corrected for. Both primary endpoints were met. The prednisolone dose could be reduced more significantly with MTX (difference –22.3 (CI –36.2 - (–5.4), p=0.010, logarithmically analyzed), and the SLAM-R was also reduced (difference –0.86 (CI –1.72 - (–0.02), p=0.039). Of the secondary endpoints, only the mental sum score of the MOS-SF-36, but not the physical sum score or the SLEDAI, reached the significance level.

In contrast, a meta-analysis of randomized controlled trials (25) also showed a significant benefit for SLE activity by SLEDAI (RR 0.444 (CI 0.279-0.707)). As expected, the steroid-sparing effect was significant (RR 0.335 (CI 0.202-0.558)).

Overall, MTX is effective in SLE, especially for the most common manifestations that are not organ-threatening, and is accordingly recommended by expert consensus (20, 26).

6.3.2. Systemic sclerosis

The EULAR recommendations (27) include MTX as a possible treatment for active skin manifestations in diffuse cutaneous systemic sclerosis (dcSSc). While the number of proven options for the treatment of SSc is very limited overall, there are at least two controlled studies for MTX (28). The 24-week study published by van den Hoogen et al. randomized 17 patients with early dcSSc to MTX (15 mg per week intramuscularly) and 12 to placebo (29). Of the 15 patients who completed the study in the MTX arm, 5 had a measurable benefit (3 in the skin score, 4 in the VAS, both in 1), but only 1/10 in the placebo arm (p=0.03). There was only a non-significant trend for the improvement of the skin score (p=0.06). In the six-month extension (15 mg per week in the 8 responders and 9 patients in the placebo group, 25 mg per week in 6 non-responders), 15/23 (68%) showed an improvement at week 48.

The second, unfortunately negative placebo-controlled trial by Pope et al. (30) also provides at least some indication of an improvement in skin involvement in dcSSc. 71 patients with dcSSc and disease duration of up to three years were randomized. The modified Rodnan skin score (mRSS) fell slightly under MTX (from 28±2 to 27±3 after 3, 25±2 after 6 and 24±2 after 12 months), while it remained the same in the placebo group (27±2, 29±2, 29±2, 29±2). 9 patients did not improve under MTX, but 10 did improve by 21-50% and 3 by 51-70%; in the placebo arm, the figures were 12, 8 and 1 patient(s), respectively. Unfortunately, there was no indication of an effect on lung involvement.

Overall, there is evidence of an effect of MTX therapy on skin involvement, while no effects on ILD were seen. Therefore, MTX represents a treatment option, especially in patients with active dcSSc (27) without active lung involvement and with arthritis associated with SSc or SSc-RA overlap syndromes.

6.3.3. Poly- and dermatomyositis

Although MTX is one of the most commonly used therapies for autoimmune myositis (31), the data is still not completely convincing, especially for adults.

The best data is available for juvenile dermatomyositis, where a randomized controlled trial conducted by the Paediatric Rheumatology International Trials Organization (PRINTO) included a total of 139 patients and randomized them to MTX (n=46), ciclosporin A (CsA) (n=46) or monotherapy with glucocorticoids (n=47) (32). After 6 months, 72% of the patients on MTX, but only 51% of those on prednisolone monotherapy, achieved a PRINTO20 improvement. The median remission with MTX was achieved after 42 months; in the other treatment arms, less than 50% achieved remission.

The data in adults is not so clear. Vencovsky et al. (33) tested MTX (7.5-15 mg per week orally, n=17) versus CsA (3.0-3.5 mg/kg, n=19) in 36 patients. This study showed no significant difference between the two arms. In a study with refractory patients, the combination of MTX (up to 25 mg per week) and AZA (150 mg) versus an oncological MTX regimen (with leucovorin rescue) (34) also showed no difference. 12 of the 58 patients included in the SELAM study were randomized to MTX and 15 to MTX and CsA, of whom 6 and 11 respectively completed one year of treatment. The CK reduction using MTX was not significant by a narrow margin (p=0.060). The negative results of the randomized PROMETHEUS study with a total of 31 patients (17 PP, 14 DM) were never fully published after their presentation in abstract form in 2014 (35). In these patients with newly onset myositis, there was no benefit in relation to the total dose of glucocorticoids when using MTX (maximum 20 mg per week) plus glucocorticoids versus monotherapy with glucocorticoids. In this context, however, it should be noted that at least for PM there is no proven therapy with immunosuppressants or synthetic or biological DMARDs (36).

Disease	Approved	Recommended	Best evidence for effectivity
Ankylosing spondylitis/ Axial spondyloarthritis	no	no (1)	None
Psoriatic arthritis	yes	yes (2, 3)	Small, only partly positive RCTs, leflunomide equivalent
Giant cell arteritis	no	alternative (11)	Positive meta-analysis of partly negative RCTs
GPA, MPA, EGPA	no	yes (15)	RCTs for induction (vs cyclophosphamide) and maintenance (vs azathioprine)
SLE	no	yes (20)	Positive meta-analysis of small positive RCTs
SSc	no	yes (26)	Non-significant trend in skin improvement in RCTs
PM/DM	no	not formally	Azathioprine and ciclosporin equivalent (RCTs)
MCTD	no	not formally	Case studies

Table 6.1: Overview of MTX in spondyloarthritides, vasculitides and connective tissue diseases.
GPA: Granulomatosis with polyangiitis (formerly: Wegener's disease); **MPA**: Microscopic polyangiitis; **EGPA**: Eosinophilic granulomatosis with polyangiitis (formerly: Churg-Strauss syndrome); **SLE**: Systemic lupus erythematosus; **SSc**: Systemic sclerosis; **PM/DM**: Polymyositis/dermatomyositis; **MCTD**: Mixed connective tissue disease, mixed connective tissue disease; **RCTs**: randomized controlled clinical trials.

6.3.4. Mixed connective tissue disease

As of 2010 (28), there are still no controlled data available on the treatment of mixed connective tissue disease (MCTD) with MTX. There are also no official recommendations. Its use, which is nevertheless sensible in many cases, is therefore based on case reports and analogous conclusions from data in the treatment of RA, SLE and myositis.

6.4. Summary

> Overall, it can be stated that MTX is part of the standard therapy repertoire for many conditions beyond RA (☞ Table 6.1).

While the lack of conclusive evidence for PsA can only be understood on the basis of its use in this area for many decades (long before the time of major RA studies), the data for the other conditions essentially corresponds at least to that of other non-biological DMARDs and immunosuppressants. Placebo-controlled studies would be desirable for all of these indications, but in most cases they no longer seem realistic, so we will continue to have to make therapeutic decisions based on suboptimal data.

6.5. References

1. van der Heijde D, Ramiro S, Landewé R, Baraliakos X, Van den Bosch F, Sepriano A, et al. 2016 update of the ASAS/EULAR recommendations for the management of ankylosing spondylitis. Ann Rheum Dis 2017;76(6): 978-991.

2. Gossec L, Kerschbaumer A, Ferreira RJO, Aletaha D, Baraliakos X, Bertheussen H et al. European League Against Rheumatism recommendations for the management of psoriatic arthritis with pharmacological therapies: 2023 update. Ann Rheum Dis 2024;83(6):706-719.

3. Coates LC, Kavanaugh A, Mease PJ, Soriano ER, Laura Acosta-Felquer M, Armstrong AW, et al. Group for Research and Assessment of Psoriasis and Psoriatic Arthritis 2015 treatment recommendations for psoriatic arthritis. Arthritis Rheumatol 2016;68(5):1060-1071.

4. Scarpa R, Peluso R, Atteno M, Manguso F, Spano A, Iervolino S et al. The effectiveness of a traditional therapeutical approach in early psoriatic arthritis: results of a pilot randomised 6-month trial with methotrexate. J Clin Rheumatol 2011; 17:169-172.

5. Kingsley GH, Kowalczyk A, Taylor H, Ibrahim F, Packham JC, McHugh NJ et al. A randomized placebo-controlled trial of MTX in PsA. Rheumatology 2012;51: 1368-1377.

6. Wilsdon TD, Whittle SL, Thynne TR, Mangoni AA. Methotrexate for psoriatic arthritis. Cochrane Database Syst Rev 2019;1(1):CD012722.

7. Coates LC, Helliwell PS. Methotrexate efficacy in the Tight Control in Psoriatic Arthritis study. J Rheumatol 2016;43(2): 356-361.

8. Combe B, Behrens F, McHugh N, Brock F, Kerkmann U, Kola B, et al. Comparison of etanercept monotherapy and combination therapy with methotrexate in psoriatic arthritis: Results from 2 clinical trials. J Rheumatol 2016; 43(6):1063-1067.

9. Behrens F, Koehm M, Schwaneck EC, Schmalzing M, Wittig BM, Gnann H, et al. Addition or removal of concomitant methotrexate alters adalimumab effectiveness in rheumatoid arthritis but not psoriatic arthritis. Scand J Rheumatol 2019; 48(5):375-382.

10. Mease PJ, Gladman DD, Collier DH, Ritchlin CT, Helliwell PS, Liu L, et al. Etanercept and methotrexate as monotherapy or in combination for psoriatic arthritis: primary results from a randomized, controlled phase III trial. Arthritis Rheumatol 2019;71(7):1112-1124.

11. Hellmich B, Agueda A, Monti S, Buttgereit F, de Boysson H, Brouwer E, et al. 2018 Update of the EULAR recommendations for the management of large vessel vasculitis. Ann Rheum Dis 2020;79(1):19-30.

12. Mahr AD, Jover JA, Spiera RF, Hernandez-Garcia C, Fernandez-Gutierrez B, Lavalley MP et al. Adjunctive methotrexate for treatment of giant cell arteritis: an individual patient data meta-analysis. Arthritis Rheum 2007; 56(8):2789-97.

13. Yates M, Loke YK, Watts RA, MacGregor AJ. Prednisolone combined with adjunctive immunosuppression is not superior to prednisolone alone in terms of efficacy and safety in giant cell arteritis: meta-analysis. Clin Rheumatol 2014;33(2): 227-36.

14. Reinhold-Keller E, de GK. Use of methotrexate in ANCA-associated vasculitides. Clin Exp Rheumatol 2010;28(5 Suppl 61):S178-S182.

15. Hellmich B, Sanchez-Alamo B, Schirmer JH, Berti A, Blockmans D, Cid MC et al. EULAR recommendations for the management of ANCA-associated vasculitis: 2022 update. Ann Rheum Dis 2024;83(1):30-47.

16. de GK, Rasmussen N, Bacon PA, Tervaert JW, Feighery C, Gregorini G et al. Randomized trial of cyclophosphamide versus methotrexate for induction of remission in early systemic antineutrophil cytoplasmic antibody-associated vasculitis. Arthritis Rheum 2005;52 (8):2461-9.

17. Faurschou M, Westman K, Rasmussen N, de GK, Flossmann O, Hoglund P et al. Brief Report: long-term outcome of a randomized clinical trial comparing methotrexate to cyclophosphamide for remission induction in early systemic antineutrophil cytoplasmic antibody-associated vasculitis. Arthritis Rheum 2012;64(10): 3472-7.

18. Pagnoux C, Mahr A, Hamidou MA, Boffa JJ, Ruivard M, Ducroix JP et al. Azathioprine or methotrexate maintenance for ANCA-associated vasculitis. N Engl J Med 2008; 359(26): 2790-803.

19. Jayne D, Rasmussen N, Andrassy K, Bacon P, Tervaert JW, Dadoniene J et al. A randomized trial of maintenance therapy for vasculitis associated with antineutrophil cytoplasmic autoantibodies. N Engl J Med 2003; 349(1):36-44.

20. Springer J, Nutter B, Langford CA, Hoffman GS, Villa-Forte A. Granulomatosis with polyangiitis (Wegener's): impact of maintenance therapy duration. Medicine 2014;93(2): 82-90.

21. Fanouriakis A, Kostopoulou M, Andersen J, Aringer M, Arnaud L, Bae SC, et al. EULAR recommendations for the management of systemic lupus erythematosus: 2023 update. Ann Rheum Dis 2024;83(1):15-29.

22. Pego-Reigosa JM, Cobo-Ibanez T, Calvo-Alen J, Loza-Santamaria E, Rahman A, Munoz-Fernandez S et al. Efficacy and safety of nonbiologic immunosuppressants in the treatment of nonrenal systemic lupus erythematosus: a systematic review. Arthritis Care Res 2013;65(11): 1775-85.

23. Winzer M, Aringer M. Use of methotrexate in patients with systemic lupus erythematosus and primary Sjogren's syndrome. Clin Exp Rheumatol 2010;28(5 Suppl 61):S156-S159.

24. Fortin PR, Abrahamowicz M, Ferland D, Lacaille D, Smith CD, Zummer M. Steroid-sparing effects of methotrexate in systemic lupus erythematosus: a double-blind, randomized, placebo-controlled trial. Arthritis Rheum 2008;59(12):1796-804.

25. Sakthiswary R, Suresh E. Methotrexate in systemic lupus erythematosus: a systematic review of its efficacy. Lupus 2014; 23(3):225-35.

26. Aringer M, Burkhardt H, Burmester GR, Fischer-Betz R, Fleck M, Graninger W et al. Current state of evidence on "off label" therapeutic options for systemic lupus erythematosus, including biological immunosuppressive agents, in Germany, Austria, and Switzerland - a consensus report. Lupus 2012; 21(4):386-401.

27. Del Galdo F, Lescoat A, Conaghan PG, Bertoldo E, ?oli? J, Santiago T et al. EULAR recommendations for the treatment of systemic sclerosis: 2023 update. Ann Rheum Dis 2024 Oct 17 Epub. doi: 10.1136/ard-2024-226430.

28. Kowal-Bielecka O, Distler O. Use of methotrexate in patients with scleroderma and mixed connective tissue disease. Clin Exp Rheumatol 2010;28(5 Suppl 61):S160-S163.

29. van den Hoogen FH, Spronk PE, Boerbooms AM, Bootsma H, de Rooij DJ, Kallenberg CG et al. Long-term follow-up of 46 patients with anti-(U1)snRNP antibodies. Br J Rheumatol 1994;33(12):1117-20.

30. Pope JE, Bellamy N, Seibold JR, Baron M, Ellman M, Carette S et al. A randomized, controlled trial of methotrexate versus placebo in early diffuse scleroderma. Arthritis Rheum 2001;44(6):1351-8.

31. Tansley S, Shaddick G, Christopher-Stine L, Sharp C, Dourmishev L, Maurer B, et al. Developing standardised treatment for adults with myositis and different phenotypes: an international survey of current prescribing preferences. Clin Exp Rheumatol 2016;34(5): 880-884.

32. Ruperto N, Pistorio A, Oliveira S, Zulian F, Cuttica R, Ravelli A, et al. Prednisone versus prednisone plus ciclosporin versus prednisone plus methotrexate in new-onset juvenile dermatomyositis: a randomised trial. Lancet 2016;387 (10019):671-678.

33. Vencovsky J, Jarosova K, Machacek S, Studynkova J, Kafkova J, Bartunkova J et al. Cyclosporine A versus methotrexate in the treatment of polymyositis and dermatomyositis. Scand J Rheumatol 2000;29(2):95-102.

34. Villalba L, Hicks JE, Adams EM, Sherman JB, Gourley MF, Leff RL et al. Treatment of refractory myositis: a randomized crossover study of two new cytotoxic regimens. Arthritis Rheum 1998;41(3):392-9.

35. Tomasova Studynkova J, Mann H, Jarosova K, Blumhardt S, Maurer B, Dastmalchi M et al. A prospective, randomized, open-label, assessor-blind, multicenter study of efficacy and safety of combined treatment of methotrextzae + glucocorticoids versus glucocorticoids alone in patients with polymyositis and dermatomyositis (PROMETHEUS trial). Ann Rheum Dis 2014;73[S2]: 171.

36. Gordon PA, Winer JB, Hoogendijk JE, Choy EH. Immunosuppressant and immunomodulatory treatment for dermatomyositis and polymyositis. Cochrane Database Syst Rev 2012;8:CD003643.

7. Methotrexate in childhood and adolescence

Methotrexate (MTX) has been the disease-modifying antirheumatic drug (DMARD) most commonly used in pediatric rheumatology since the 1990s.

> MTX is the DMARD of choice for juvenile idiopathic arthritis (JIA).
> - In 2020, almost half of the approximately 7,000 JIA patients recorded in the (national pediatric rheumatology) database received MTX.
> - Among patients with polyarthritis, it was two thirds.

However, MTX is also the preferred DMARD for other juvenile rheumatic diseases, e.g.

- juvenile dermatomyositis,
- linear scleroderma or
- idiopathic uveitis.

In view of the main area of application of MTX and the available evidence, this chapter is limited to the use of MTX in JIA and JIA-associated uveitis. The type of application (e.g. dose, mode of application) and the side effect profile are not fundamentally different when used beyond JIA.

7.1. Efficacy in juvenile idiopathic arthritis

Several randomized controlled and open prospective studies have demonstrated the efficacy of MTX in JIA (☞ Table 7.1). The patient groups studied were heterogeneous; they mainly included patients with polyarticular JIA. The study periods in the randomized controlled trials (RCTs) were relatively short, ranging from 3 to 12 months. The therapeutic success was generally assessed using the ACR Ped response criteria proposed in 1997 (7) or the proportion of patients with clinically inactive disease (according to the Wallace criteria (8)). Based on the available data, approximately two thirds of children and adolescents with JIA respond to MTX at a dose of 10-20 mg/m² body surface area (BSA) per week, i.e. these patients improve by at least 30% in at least three clinical parameters and achieve a ACR Ped-30 response (7). The desired therapeutic goal, clinically inactive disease (8), is achieved by between 20-35% of patients in RCTs after 12 months of treatment. The rates are higher in observational studies. Based on data from the Canadian JIA early cohort ReACCh-Out, a response rate to MTX (possibly in combination with NSAIDs and/or intra-articular glucocorticoids) of 60% was determined, i.e. the patients achieved clinically inactive, or at least minimally active, disease (9).

MTX is the preferred DMARD for combination treatment with biological DMARDs (bDMARDs). The extent to which it increases the efficacy of bDMARDs is not well documented for JIA. At least in the adalimumab (ADA) approval study, the ACR Ped-30, -50 and -70 response rates were higher in patients who received ADA in combination with MTX than in patients with ADA monotherapy (10). In addition, MTX reduces the risk of developing anti-drug antibodies and thus the risk of secondary drug failure in monoclonal TNF antibody therapy.

JIA includes various diseases with different treatment responses. Although most of the available studies could not determine any influence of the JIA category on the MTX response (11), the relatively small number of patients in the various JIA categories in these studies must be taken into account. Patients with *extended oligoarthritis* respond particularly well to MTX, whereas patients with systemic onset of JIA respond less well than patients with oligoarthritis or polyarthritis (2). In view of data from the JIA biologics registers and internal rheumatology, it can also be assumed that MTX is less effective in psoriatic arthritis (PsA) and that MTX is only effective to a limited extent in enthesitis-related arthritis, especially in cases of axial involvement.

In patients with polyarticular JIA, symptoms of the disease subside after initiating MTX therapy. Disease activity (including the number of active and restricted joints) decreases significantly, and the patients' functional ability and growth improve. The patients' quality of life, especially their physical health, also improves (☞ Figure 7.1).

Author	Design	Patient number	MTX dosage per week	Patient collective	*Follow-up*	Response
Giannini et al., 1992 [1]	RCT	127	5 or 10 mg/m² BSA PO	20% OA 51% Poly 29% sJIA	6 mo	Special Composite Index: • 10 mg MTX 63% • 5 mg MTX 32% • Placebo 36%
Ruperto et al., 1998	open, prospective	111	10 mg/m² BSA PO	20% OA 51% Poly 29% sJIA	6 mo	ACR Ped-30: 66%
Woo et al., 2000 [2]	RCT	88	15-20 mg/m² BSA PO	49% extOA 51% sJIA	4 mo	Modified ACR Ped-30 (based on 5 criteria): • sysJIA: MTX 25% vs placebo 16% • ext OA: MTX 48% vs placebo 18%
Ruperto et al., 2004 [3]	open, prospective	595	8-12,5 mg/m² BSA PO, SC, IM	31% extOA 55% Poly 15% sJIA	6 mo	• ACR Ped-30: 72% • ACR Ped-70: 38% • Inactive disease: 12%
	RCT	80 non-responders	15 mg/m² BSA (max. 20 mg) vs 30 mg/m² BSA (max. 40 mg) SC, IM	29% extOA 55% Poly 16% sJIA	6 mo	ACR Ped-30: • 15 mg/m² BSA: 62,5% • 30 mg/m² BSA: 57,5% Ped-ACR-70: • 15 mg/m² BSA: 45% • 30 mg/m² BSA: 47,5% Inactive disease: • 15 mg/m² BSA: 12,5% • 30 mg/m² BSA: 10%
Tynjäla et al., 2011 (4)	RCT	20	15 mg/m² BSA (max. 25 mg)	75% Poly 20% EAA 5% PsA	54 wks	• ACR Ped-75: 50% • Inactive disease: 25%
Wallace et al., 2012 [5]	RCT (MTX open)	43	0,5 mg/kg (max. 40 mg) SC	100% Poly	4 mo	• ACR Ped-70: 44%
					12 mo	• Inactive disease: 16%
Hissink Muller et al., 2017	RCT (Best for Kids)	32 (MTX + 6 wks prednisolone)	10 mg/m² BSA (max. 25 mg)	9% OA 69% Poly 22% PsA	3 mo	• ACR Ped-70: 19% • Inactive disease: 9%
Ravelli et al., 2017 [6]	randomized, open	105 (MTX and IA GC)	15 mg/m² BSA (max. 25 mg) PO	100% OA	12 mo	• Inactive disease: 36%
Alexeeva et al., 2021	RCT	33 (MTX arm)	10-15 mg	36% extOA 48% Poly 9% EAA 6% other JIA	3 mo 6 mo 12 mo	• ACR Ped-30: 61% • Inactive disease: 27% • Inactive disease: 21%

Table 7.1: Selected studies on the effectivity of MTX. **OA** = oligoarthritis; **extOA** = extended oligoarthritis; **Poly** = polyarthritis (rheumatoid factor positive or negative); **EAA** = enthesitis-associated arthritis; **PsA** = psoriatic arthritis; **sJIA** = systemic JIA; **GC** = glucocorticoids; **wks** = weeks; **mo** = months; **PO** = oral; **SC** = subcutaneous; **IM** = intramuscular; **BSA** = body surface area; **RCT** = randomized controlled trial.

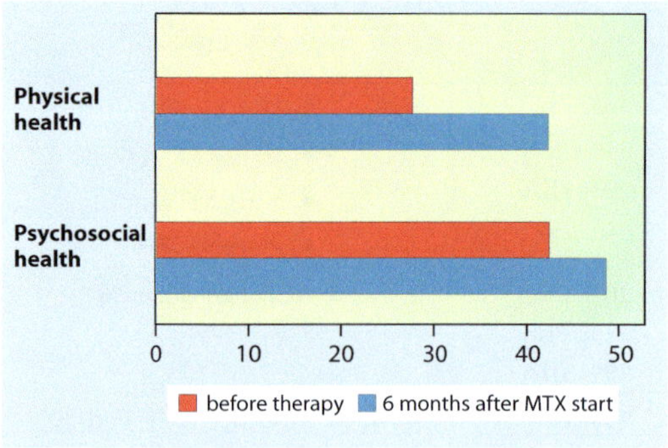

Figure 7.1: Quality of life of 521 children with JIA assessed using the Child Health Questionnaire (standardized sum scores) before and 6 months after starting MTX therapy. Modified from Céspedes-Cruz et al, 2006 (12).

The extent to which MTX can prevent or halt radiographic joint changes in children with JIA was not examined in RCTs. It was shown that MTX therapy can also prevent radiographic progression in a treat-to-target approach (13). In order to halt or prevent structural joint damage, at least a ACR Ped-90 response is required.

MTX is approved for the treatment of polyarticular JIA in children from the age of 2 years. Its use is recommended if NSAIDs and/or intra-articular glucocorticoids have not led to therapeutic success (14-16). In persistent oligoarthritis, MTX must still be used off-label despite appropriate treatment recommendations.

There is increasing evidence that early attainment of inactive disease improves the prognosis of JIA. Therefore, a treat-to-target approach is recommended: in polyarticular JIA, MTX therapy is commenced immediately after diagnosis and treatment is escalated after 3 or 6 months if the desired treatment goal has not been achieved (17).

7.2. Juvenile idiopathic arthritis-associated uveitis

MTX is also the first-line DMARD in the treatment of uveitis, although its effectivity has not yet been demonstrated in a randomized controlled trial. In the published retrospective case series, response rates were between 50 and 85%, although the treatment response was assessed using different methods. In the meta-analysis by Simonini et al., which included nine studies in which the majority of patients had JIA-associated uveitis, a response rate of 73% was determined (18). MTX is recommended for JIA-associated uveitis if topical corticosteroids do not resolve the inflammation within 3 months or if new complications arise (19, 20). In a randomized controlled trial, the efficacy of ADA in combination with MTX in anterior non-infectious uveitis was demonstrated (21).

If children and adolescents are treated with MTX because of joint symptoms, they have a lower risk of developing uveitis. There is also a lower risk of uveitis in children who are treated early with MTX in combination with a TNF blocker. Uveitis is particularly rare in combination therapy with MTX + ADA.

However, MTX is not approved as monotherapy for the treatment of active anterior uveitis in children with JIA.

7.3. Predictors of treatment response in juvenile idiopathic arthritis

A meta-analysis of 20 studies identified possible predictors of treatment response to MTX (11). Predictors of treatment response include higher disease activity (global assessment by physician), higher serum concentrations of S100A8/A9 proteins at the start of treatment, and ANA positivity. A poorer treatment response is associated with wrist involvement, a longer duration of disease, and a higher degree of functional impairment at the start of treatment. Other interesting parameters with predictive value for treatment response are intracellular concentrations of long-chain MTX polyglutamates, the serum concentration of the pro-inflammatory molecule osteopontin, and the hemoglobin concentration (11).

Gene variants that affect the absorption, distribution, metabolism and excretion of the drug, for example through changes in enzyme properties, probably also influence the response to MTX. The CHARMS (Sparks Childhood Arthritis Response to Medication Study) cohort showed that single nucleotide polymorphisms (SNPs) in the *ATIC* (5-aminoimidazole-4-carboxamide ribonucleotide formyltransferase/IMP cyclohydrolase) gene are associated with a lower response to MTX, possibly

ACR Ped Response [Giannini et al., 1997]	
ACR Ped-30 Response: Improvement of at least 30% in at least 3 of the 6 core set parameters listed below and deterioration of >30% in a maximum of one parameter. **ACR Ped-50/70/90/100 Response:** Improvement of at least 50/70/90/100% in at least 3 of the 6 core set parameters and deterioration of >30% in a maximum of one parameter.	
1.	Global assessment of disease activity by the doctor (e.g. using a numerical rating scale [NRS] or visual analogue scale [VAS])
2.	Global assessment of general well-being by the patient or his/her parents (e.g. using NRS or VAS)
3.	Number of joints with active arthritis
4.	Number of joints with restricted movement
5.	Functioning in everyday life (e.g. using the Childhood Health Assessment Questionnaire [CHAQ])
6.	Acute phase parameters (ESR or CrP)
Clinically inactive disease (in the case of persistent or extended oligoarthritis, rheumatoid factor negative or positive polyarthritis and systemic onset JIA) [Wallace et al., 2011]: The following criteria must apply • No active arthritis • No fever, no rash, no serositis, no splenomegaly or generalized lymph node swelling as a result of JIA • No active uveitis (based on the definition of the Standardization of Uveitis Nomenclature) • Normal ESR or normal CRP (if elevated, not due to JIA) • Best possible value in terms of the global assessment of disease activity by the physician • Morning stiffness ≤15 minutes	
Remission *with* therapy = inactive disease for at least 6 months	
Remission *without* therapy = inactive disease for at least 12 months without any antirheumatic therapy	

Table 7.2: Definition of treatment success in JIA using the ACR Ped response.

through a reduction in adenosine production. A Dutch study showed that SNPs in two transporter genes (*ABCB1* and *ABCC3*) increase the likelihood of a good response within the first year of treatment, and a SNP in another transporter gene (*SLC19A1*) reduces the likelihood of a response by a factor of 2-3. *SLC19A1* transports MTX into the cell, *ABCB1* and *ABCC3* out of the cell, i.e. variations in these genes probably influence the intracellular MTX concentration (11). However, a reliable specific genetic marker to predict the efficacy of MTX has not yet been identified (22).

Based on clinical and genetic predictors, a prediction model for non-response to MTX therapy (failure to achieve ACR Ped-70 in the first year of treatment) was developed. It takes into account the ESR and SNPs of 4 genes (*MTRR* [methionine synthase reductase], *MDR-1/ABCB1* [multi drug resistance 1], *MRP-1/ABCC1* [multi drug resistance protein 1] and *PCFT* [proton-coupled folate transporter] gene). In two JIA validation cohorts, 72% and 65% of patients were correctly classified, respectively (23). Further validation of the model is required before it can be recommended for practice.

Most of the predictors mentioned were only found in one study and confirmation is pending. A practical, reliable prediction model does not yet exist. However, it is undoubtedly proven that the time between the onset of symptoms and the start of treatment determines the response, i.e. the shorter the time period, the greater the likelihood of a response to MTX. With each year until the start of treatment with MTX, the chance of achieving an inactive disease is reduced by 17% (9). If patients respond to MTX within the first three or six months of treatment, a good treatment effect can be expected after 12 months or five years.

7.4. Dosage and form of administration of methotrexate in pediatric rheumatology

MTX is usually administered subcutaneously or orally at a dose of (10) to 15 to (20) mg/m² BSA per week. An MTX dose of 5 mg/m² BSA per week is not associated with a demonstrable effect compared to placebo (1). Doses above 20 mg/m² BSA per week do not lead to any further increase in the effectivity of MTX (3).

> The recommended starting dose is around 15 mg/m² body weight per week (9).

The bioavailability after oral administration is subject to large interindividual variability. Absorption is usually poorer at higher doses, which is why parenteral administration is preferred from 15 mg/m² BSA. Whether taking MTX on an empty stomach improves bioavailability has not been proven beyond doubt. At least a small study on children with JIA suggests this.

The better efficacy of parenteral administration has not yet been proven in children, but a randomized study has not been conducted. However, more than half of the non-responders to oral MTX respond to treatment when they are switched to subcutaneous administration (3). For the treatment of uveitis, subcutaneous administration is recommended before oral administration (20). MTX is often given with folic acid (5 mg approximately 24 hours after taking MTX) to avoid side effects such as nausea, stomatitis or elevated liver values. The effectivity of MTX is not affected by this.

7.5. Tolerability of methotrexate

> MTX is a relatively safe substance for long-term use in children and adolescents.

It very rarely leads to serious toxic side effects. However, adverse events (AEs) possibly related to MTX are reported in at least half of the patients (☞ Table 7.3) (24). Gastrointestinal complaints with nausea, vomiting and abdominal pain occur most frequently within 24 to 48 hours after ingestion. Gastrointestinal complaints are part of the symptom complex of subjective MTX "intolerance", which is the main problem in long-term use of MTX. The intolerance affects more than half of the patients and is subject to conditioning, so that anticipatory nausea can occur even before MTX is taken. The intolerance can be quantified using the Methotrexate Intolerance Severity Score (MISS) (values ≥6 are considered relevant) and often begins in the first year of therapy. It usually increases with the further duration of therapy. There is currently no effective strategy to combat this side effect; attempts include changing the MTX application form, evening medication administration before/on the weekend, cognitive behavioral therapies, the administration of antiemetics and pharmacological conditioning (24).

In addition, mild and transient elevations in transaminases are often observed, i.e. in about a third of patients. In up to 5% of cases (not significantly more often than in patients not treated with MTX), they exceed twice the upper limit of normal, more frequently in patients with systemic JIA. Laboratory tests during MTX use are therefore recommended less frequently in children and adolescents than in adults, namely once within the first 4-8 weeks after starting and then every 3-4 months (16). In the future, treatment monitoring based on the patient's individual risk profile (defined, for example, by certain gene variants) is conceivable. Whether intraerythrocytic polyglutamate concentrations of MTX are suitable for this remains to be proven. To date, the data regarding the risk of gastrointestinal and hepatotoxic side effects associated with certain concentrations of MTX polyglutamates are contradictory.

Furthermore, stomatitis (10%), hair loss (5%) and leukocytopenia (≤4,000/mm³ in 5%) have been reported in children taking MTX (3). Pulmonary toxicity is very rare. Two cases of MTX pneumonitis in JIA patients have been published so far (☞ also Chapter 10.4.).

In principle, MTX does not seem to significantly increase the risk of infections in children and adolescents. An analysis of health insurance data found that JIA patients treated with MTX did not have a significantly higher risk of serious infections, i.e. infections leading to hospitalization, compared to those not treated with MTX. However, JIA patients have a higher background risk of serious and opportunistic infections. It is therefore recommended that vaccination status be completed, particularly for varicella, before starting (MTX) therapy and that the annual flu vaccination be given. Inactivated vaccines can be administered without restriction under MTX. Some studies, including a randomized one, have demonstrated the immunogenicity and tolerability of live vaccines in JIA patients receiving MTX (25). VZV primary vaccination and MMR booster vaccinations can therefore be considered in patients receiving MTX at a standard dose of ≤15 mg/m² BSA.

Isolated case reports of malignant diseases in patients treated with MTX, particularly lymphomas – some of which are EBV-associated – have been published. It is possible that these are at least partially attributable to the background risk of malignant diseases in JIA.

MTX does not affect fertility, but is potentially teratogenic. Therefore, adolescents should be advised on safe contraception.

Predictors have also been identified for the occurrence of MTX-related AEs in general or for specific AEs such as liver toxicity, gastrointestinal complaints or MTX intolerance (11). However, the data situation is even more limited than for the predictors of MTX response. Interesting predictor candidates are increases in alanine aminotransferase, platelet count, the JIA category polyarthritis and gene variants in the *GGH* (γ-glutamyl hydroxylase, involved in the degradation of MTX polyglutamates) and *MTHFR* (methylenetetrahydrofolate reductase, involved in folic acid metabolism) genes. However, reliable predictive genetic markers do not yet exist [22].

The Dutch working group led by Dijkhuizen developed a first prediction model for MTX intolerance based on seven clinical parameters. If none of the seven clinical predictors is present, the risk of MTX intolerance is 19%; if all of them are present (polyarthritis, ANA positivity, pain intensity of 3-6 [on NRS], JADAS-27 ≤5, platelet count >350 Gpt/l, ALT ≤12 IU/l and creatinine ≤50 μmol/l) the risk of intolerance is 86%. With an overall risk value of ≥6, the sensitivity of the model was 82% and the specificity 56%. Validation in an independent cohort is pending (11).

7.6. Adherence to therapy

MTX is usually administered to JIA patients over a period of several years. Long-term therapy is made difficult by the frequency of MTX intolerance, which impairs adherence to therapy.

An analysis of health insurance data from 1,964 children revealed an MTX treatment adherence of around 50% within one year of observation, with adherence being better for oral than for subcutaneous administration and better for children under 13 years than for adolescents. In a smaller study, adherence to therapy was over 80%, but was based only on information provided by parents during consultations. The main reason for not taking the medication was the child's refusal to take the medication.

The average duration of treatment for the first MTX application in children and adolescents with JIA is less than 3 years (median), and that of a second MTX course is less than 2 years. The most common reasons for discontinuation in the first years of treatment are insufficient therapeutic effect, remission and adverse events, each occurring in about one third of cases (23). The longer the duration of treatment, the higher the rate of treatment discontinuation due to MTX intolerance.

After discontinuation of MTX therapy, arthritis or JIA-associated uveitis recurs in at least 50% of cases. According to a European randomized study, the time spent with inactive disease before discontinuation (6 months versus 12 months) plays no role in the risk of recurrence. The level of the serum concentration of S100A8/9 proteins, on the other hand, is predictive of an arthritis flare within the next 3 months (26). In contrast, retrospective studies have shown that uveitis recurrence occurs significantly less frequently if MTX is only discontinued after more than three years of treatment or after more than two years of inactive uveitis (14, 15). Whether the risk of recurrence after MTX discontinuation is lower if MTX is initially slowly reduced in dose before discontinuation or is given at longer intervals (e.g. every other week) has not been systematically investigated. If MTX is given in combination with a TNF inhibitor, the risk of recurrence within 4 years is lower; MTX is discontinued first and then the TNF inhibitor.

Author/ year	Design	Pat. no.	MTX dosage per week	Patient collective	*Fol-low-up*	Events
Giannini et al., 1992 (1)	RCT	127	5 or 10 mg/m² BSA PO	20% OA (Beginn) 51 % Poly 29 % sJIA	6 mo	• AEs in 13% (10 mg MTX), 20% (5 mg MTX) and 12% (placebo) of patients • Most common AE: gastro-intestinal complaints (50% with MTX, 100% with place-bo)
Ruperto et al., 2004 (3)	RCT	80	15 mg/m² BSA (max. 20 mg) vs 30 mg/m² BSA (max. 40 mg) SC, IM	29% extOA 55% Poly 16% sJIA	6 mo	• No significant differences in AE between dose groups • Most common nausea (in 21%) and vomiting (in 11%)
Giannini et al., 2009	open, prospec-tive	197	≈ 0,3 mg/kg (max. 1 mg/kg)	93% Poly 7% sJIA	36 mo	• 18.3 AE/100PY • Most common AE: elevated liver enzymes (2.1/100PY) • 4.6 SAE/100PY • 1.3 medically significant infec-tions/100PY
Becker et al., 2010	retro-spective	220	*low dose* ≤0,5 mg/kg *high dose* >0,5 mg/kg	24% OA 45% Poly 8% EAA 7% PsA 15% sJIA	6 mo	• 33% of patients with elevated liver enzymes (44% high dose vs 17% low dose)
Klein et al., 2012	open, prospec-tive	411	0,4 mg/kg PO vs 0,42 mg/kg SC	33% persOA 10% extOA 26% Poly 12% EAA 11% PsA 4% sJIA	6 mo	• 22% (MTX oral) and 27% (MTX parenteral) of patients had at least one AE • Most common gastrointestinal symptoms (53% and 41%) • 19 (PO) and 29 (SC) AE/100PY • 0.8 (PO) or 1 (SC) SAE/100PY
Kazamia et al., 2013	retro-spective	94	≤15 mg/m² BSA	22% persOA 11% extOA 24% Poly 18% EAA 9% PsA 4% sJIA	8,6 yrs	• 28% of patients at least one AE • most common nausea (50% of all AE, more common with SC administration), liver function test elevations (26%)
Klotsche et al., 2015	open, prospec-tive	1.055	n.s.	12% extOA 42% Poly 18% EAA 18% PsA 5% sJIA	2.907 PY	• 2.6 SAE/100PY • 0.5 medically significant infec-tions per 100PY
Van Dijk-huizen et al., 2015	open, prospec-tive	142	10 mg/m² BSA	41% OA 42% Poly	1 year	• Within the first year of therapy 41.5% of patients MTX intole-rant (MISS ≥6)

Table 7.3: Selected studies on the tolerability of MTX. **OA**: oligoarthritis at the onset of the disease; **persOA**: persistent oligoarthritis; **extOA**: extended oligoarthritis; **Poly**: polyarthritis; **EAA**: enthesitis-associated arthritis; **PsA**: psoriatic arthritis; **sJIA**: systemic JIA; **wks**: weeks; **mo**: months; **yrs**: years; **PO**: oral; **SC**: subcutaneous; **IM**: intramuscular; **BSA**: body surface area; **n.s.**: not specified, **RCT**: randomized controlled trial; **YoE**: years of exposure; **AE**: adverse events; **AE/100PY**: adverse events per 100 years; **SAE**: serious adverse events; **MISS**: Methotrexate Intolerance Severity Score.

The response to re-initiation of MTX therapy is generally good; around 40% of patients achieve inactive disease again within 12 months after restarting therapy.

7.7. References

Selection, complete literature available from the author

1. Giannini EH, Brewer EJ, Kuzmina N, Shaikov A, Maximov A, Vorontsov I, et al. Methotrexate in resistant juvenile rheumatoid arthritis. Results of the U.S.A.-U.S.S.R. double-blind, placebo-controlled trial. The Pediatric Rheumatology Collaborative Study Group and The Cooperative Children's Study Group. N Engl J Med. 1992;326(16):1043-9.

2. Woo P, Southwood TR, Prieur AM, Doré CJ, Grainger J, David J, et al. Randomized, placebo-controlled, crossover trial of low-dose oral methotrexate in children with extended oligoarticular or systemic arthritis. Arthritis Rheum. 2000; 43(8):1849-57.

3. Ruperto N, Murray KJ, Gerloni V, Wulffraat N, de Oliveira SK, Falcini F, et al.; Pediatric Rheumatology International Trials Organization. A randomized trial of parenteral methotrexate comparing an intermediate dose with a higher dose in children with juvenile idiopathic arthritis who failed to respond to standard doses of methotrexate. Arthritis Rheum. 2004;50(7):2191-201.

4. Tynjälä P, Vähäsalo P, Tarkiainen M, Kröger L, Aalto K, Malin M, et al. Aggressive combination drug therapy in very early polyarticular juvenile idiopathic arthritis (ACUTE-JIA): a multicentrerandomised open-label clinical trial. Ann Rheum Dis. 2011;70(9):1605-12.

5. Wallace CA, Giannini EH, Spalding SJ, Hashkes PJ, O'Neil KM, Zeft AS, et al.; Childhood Arthritis and Rheumatology Research Alliance. Trial of early aggressive therapy in polyarticular juvenile idiopathic arthritis. Arthritis Rheum. 2012; 64(6):2012-21.

6. Ravelli A, Davì S, Bracciolini G, Pistorio A, Consolaro A, van Dijkhuizen EHP, et al.; Italian Pediatric Rheumatology Study Group. Intra-articular corticosteroids versus intra-articular corticosteroids plus methotrexate in oligoarticular juvenile idiopathic arthritis: a multicentre, prospective, randomised, open-label trial. Lancet. 2017; 389(10072):909-916.

7. Giannini EH, Ruperto N, Ravelli A, Lovell DJ, Felson DT, Martini A. Preliminary definition of improvement in juvenile arthritis. Arthritis Rheum. 1997;40(7):1202-9.

8. Wallace CA, Giannini EH, Huang B, Itert L, Ruperto N; Childhood Arthritis Rheumatology Research Alliance; Pediatric Rheumatology Collaborative Study Group; Paediatric Rheumatology International Trials Organisation. American College of Rheumatology provisional criteria for defining clinical inactive disease in select categories of juvenile idiopathic arthritis. Arthritis Care Res (Hoboken). 2011;63(7):929-36.

9. Chhabra A, Oen K, Huber AM, Shiff NJ, Boire G, Benseler SM, et al.; ReACCh-Out Investigators. Real-world effectiveness of common treatment strategies for juvenileidiopathic arthritis: Results from a Canadian Cohort. Arthritis Care Res (Hoboken). 2020;72(7):897-906.

10. Lovell DJ, Ruperto N, Goodman S, Reiff A, Jung L, Jarosova K, et al. Pediatric Rheumatology Collaborative Study Group; Pediatric Rheumatology International Trials Organisation. Adalimumab with or without methotrexate in juvenile rheumatoid arthritis. N Engl J Med. 2008;359(8):810-20.

11. van Dijkhuizen EH, Wulffraat NM. Prediction of methotrexate efficacy and adverse events in patients with juvenile idiopathic arthritis: a systematic literature review. Pediatr-Rheumatol Online J. 2014;12:51.

12. Céspedes-Cruz A, Gutiérrez-Suárez R, Pistorio A, Ravelli A, Loy A, Murray KJ, et al. Pediatric Rheumatology International Trials Organization (PRINTO). Methotrexate improves the health-related quality of life of children with juvenile idiopathic arthritis. Ann Rheum Dis. 2008;67(3):309-14.

13. Hissink Muller PCE, van Braak WG, Schreurs D, Nusman CM, Bergstra SA, Hemke R, et al. No radiographic wrist damage after treatment to target in recent-onset juvenile idiopathic arthritis. Pediatr Rheumatol Online J. 2019;17(1):62.

14. S2k-Leitlinie Therapie der Juvenilen Idiopathischen Arthritis (3. Auflage, 2019). Hrsg. Gesellschaft für Kinder- und Jugendrheumatologie (GKJR) und Deutsche Gesellschaft für Kinder- und Jugendmedizin (DGKJ). Koordinatoren: Oommen PT, Schütz C. https://www. awmf.org/uploads/tx_szleitlinien/027-020l_S2k_Juvenile_Idiopathische_Arthritis_2020-10.pdf

15. Ringold S, et al. 2019 American College of Rheumatology/Arthritis Foundation Guideline for the Treatment of Juvenile Idiopathic Arthritis: Therapeutic Approaches for Non-Systemic Polyarthritis, Sacroiliitis, and Enthesitis. Arthritis Rheumatol. 2019;71:846-863.

16. Onel KB, Horton DB, Lovell DJ, Shenoi S, Cuello CA, Angeles-Han ST, et al. 2021 American College of Rheumatology Guideline for the Treatment of Juvenile Idiopathic Arthritis: Recommendations for Nonpharmacologic Therapies, Medication Monitoring, Immunizations, and Imaging. Arthritis Care Res (Hoboken) 2022.

17. Horneff G, Klein A, Ganser G, Sailer-Höck M, Günther A, Foeldvari I, Weller-Heinemann F. Protocols on classification, monitoring and therapy in children's rheumatology (PRO-KIND): results of the working group Polyarticular juvenile idiopathic arthritis. PediatrRheumatol Online J. 2017; 15(1):78.

18. Simonini G, Paudyal P, Jones GT, Cimaz R, Macfarlane GJ. Current evidence of methotrexate efficacy in childhood chronic uveitis: a systematic review and meta-analysis approach. Rheumatology 2013; 52(5):825-31.

19. S2K-Leitlinie Diagnostik und antientzündliche Therapie der Uveitis bei juveniler idiopathischer Arthritis. Stand: 03.05.2021. Hrsg. Deutsche Ophthalmologische Gesellschaft (DOG) und Gesellschaft für Kinder- und Jugendrheumatologie (GKJR). Koordinator Heiligenhaus A. https://www.awmf.org/uploads/tx_szleitlinien/045-012l_S2k_Diagnostik-anti entzuendliche-Therapie-Uveitis-juveniler-idiopathischer-Arthritis_2021-06.pdf

20. Angeles-Han ST, Ringold S, Beukelman T, Lovell D, Cuello CA, Becker ML, et al. 2019 American College of Rheumatology/Arthritis Foundation Guideline for the Screening, Monitoring, and Treatment of Juvenile Idiopathic Arthritis-Associated Uveitis. Arthritis Care Res (Hoboken). 2019;71(6):703-716.

21. Ramanan AV, Dick AD, Jones AP, McKay A, Williamson PR, Compeyrot-Lacassagne S, et al. SYCAMORE Study Group. Adalimumab plus Methotrexate for Uveitis in Juvenile Idiopathic Arthritis. N Engl J Med. 2017;376(17):1637-1646.

22. Selvestrel D, Lucafò M, Pugnetti L, Pagarin S, Moressa V, Pastore S, et al. Responses of patients with juvenile idiopathic arthritis to methotrexate: a genomic outlook. Expert Rev Clin Immunol. 2021;17(10):1131-1142.

23. Bulatovic M, Heijstek MW, Van Dijkhuizen EH, Wulffraat NM, Pluijm SM, de Jonge R. Prediction of clinical non-response to methotrexate treatment in juvenile idiopathic arthritis. Ann Rheum Dis. 2012;71(9): 1484-9.

24. Hügle B, van Dijkhuizen EHP. MTX intolerance in children and adolescents with juvenile idiopathic arthritis. Rheumatology (Oxford). 2020;59(7):1482-1488.

25. Heijstek MW, Kamphuis S, Armbrust W, Swart J, Gorter S, de Vries LD, et al. Effects of the live attenuated measles-mumps-rubella booster vaccination on disease activity in patients with juvenile idiopathic arthritis: a randomized trial. JAMA. 2013;309(23):2449-56.

26. Foell D, Wulffraat N, Wedderburn LR, Wittkowski H, Frosch M, Gerss J, et al. Paediatric Rheumatology International Trials Organization (PRINTO). Methotrexate withdrawal at 6 vs 12 months in juvenile idiopathic arthritis in remission: a randomized clinical trial. JAMA. 2010;303(13):1266-73.

8. Methotrexate for dermatological indications

8.1. Mechanisms of action of methotrexate in the skin

The mechanism of action of methotrexate (MTX) in the skin has not been elucidated to date. Various effects of MTX are known at the molecular level: the inhibitory effect on the enzyme dihydrofolate reductase and on the enzymes thymidilate synthase, 5-aminoimidazole-4-carboxamidoadenosine ribonucleotide (AICAR) transformylase and amidophosphoribosyltransferase (1). These enzymes fulfil functions in the synthesis of pyrimidine and purine bases as the basic building blocks of DNA. The lack of these building blocks caused by enzyme inhibition results in a general inhibition of cell proliferation.

In addition, MTX has pronounced anti-inflammatory activity. This can be explained in part by the inhibition of lymphocyte proliferation and the induction of apoptosis in activated T cells (1, 2). It is also known that methotrexate can regulate the production of pro-inflammatory cytokines and arachidonic acid derivatives in mononuclear inflammatory cells and neutrophils and prevent systemic macrophage activation.

Another indirect inhibition of MTX on inflammatory processes apparently results from the inhibition of the enzyme AICAR transformylase. This leads to the accumulation of AICAR and its metabolites intracellularly, thereby inhibiting the enzymes of adenosine metabolism adenosine deaminase and AMP deaminase. As a result, adenosine accumulates intracellularly and extracellularly in tissues (3). Adenosine is a specific ligand of the purinergic receptors A1-A3 (adenosine receptors 1-3). These are found on inflammatory cells and can influence their functions by regulating GTP-binding proteins. It is assumed that anti-inflammatory effects of MTX are at least partially mediated by accumulation of adenosine in inflamed tissue.

8.2. Methotrexate in the treatment of psoriasis vulgaris

8.2.1. Methotrexate as monotherapy for chronic plaque psoriasis

From the above-mentioned pharmacodynamic properties of MTX, the following mechanisms of action can be derived for the treatment of hyperproliferative inflammatory skin diseases such as psoriasis:

1. Slowing down of the pathologically increased keratinocyte proliferation in the psoriatic epidermis by inhibiting DNA synthesis
2. Inhibition of proliferation and stimulation of apoptosis of T lymphocytes and macrophages
3. Inhibition of the activation of macrophages and the formation of inflammatory mediators
4. Inhibition of the migration of inflammatory cells into inflamed tissue

It is unclear to what extent the individual mechanisms contribute to the antipsoriatic effect of MTX. It is quite possible that MTX effects are caused by a combination of several mechanisms of action.

Although MTX has been used to treat psoriasis for almost 50 years, the amount of reliable data on clinical efficacy is limited compared to other systemic therapeutics. The use of folic acid antagonists to treat psoriasis dates back to the 1950s. Initially, aminopterin was used. MTX, the successor to aminopterin, was approved for the treatment of psoriasis in the USA in 1971. It was not approved for the treatment of rheumatoid arthritis (RA) until 1988.

☞ also Chapter 1.2.

The initial observation of the clinical efficacy of MTX as a therapeutic agent for psoriasis was subsequently supported by numerous publications (4, 5). A systematic review of five systemic treatment methods for psoriasis from 1997 identified 101 published studies on the efficacy of MTX in psoriasis. None of these met the methodological requirements for inclusion in the treatment efficacy calculations performed in this study (6). A multicenter, double-blind, placebo-controlled study published in 2017 investigated the effectivity of subcutaneously administered MTX at a dosage of 17.5-22.5 mg. The primary endpoint was the PASI 75 response (a 75% improvement in the skin compared to baseline). This was achieved by 41% of patients in the verum group and 10% of patients in the placebo group. However, the limitation of this study is the small number of participants, with 91 patients in the MTX group and 29 patients in the placebo group (7).

Since MTX is still one of the most commonly used therapeutic agents for psoriasis vulgaris, so-called real-world data can be used to assess its effectivity. The effectivity of oral and subcutaneous MTX was compared using data from PsoBest, the largest psoriasis registry in German-speaking countries. Patients with moderate or severe psoriasis who had received MTX for at least 12 months at the index time were included. The PASI 90 response (a 90% reduction in skin involvement) was achieved after 52 weeks by 29.3% of patients with subcutaneous treatment and by 16% of patients with oral treatment. However, the PASI-90 treatment response after 12 weeks showed no significant difference between oral and subcutaneous administration (20.0 vs 20.3% of patients). These results may be explained, among other reasons, by a more favorable side effect profile for subcutaneous administration (8).

Overall, however, different studies show partly different results in regard to the superiority of subcutaneous administration over oral administration. Therefore, from the authors' point of view, the decision on the administration route can be made on a case-by-case basis.

8.2.2. Methotrexate for other forms of psoriasis

8.2.2.1. Pustular psoriasis and nail psoriasis

There are no controlled studies on the use of MTX in the treatment of pustular psoriasis, neither for the generalized variant, nor for the form localized on the hands and feet (palmoplantar pustular psoriasis) or nail psoriasis (☞ Figure 8.1). Nevertheless, MTX is used successfully in individual cases in everyday clinical practice, particularly for the localized form. This also applies to the rare variant of pustular psoriasis, acrodermatitis continua Hallopeau.

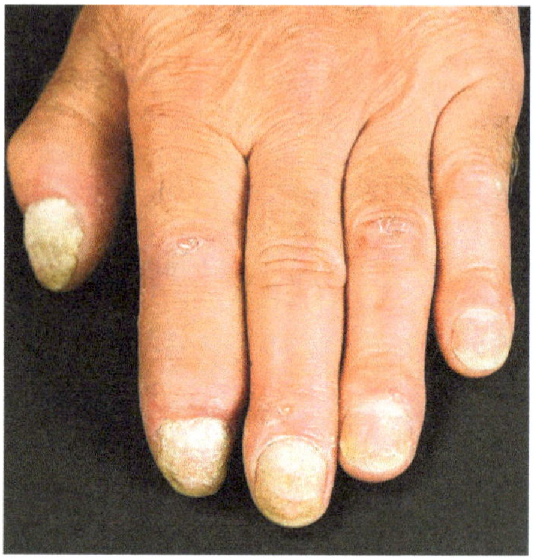

Figure 8.1: Psoriatic nail changes.

Several literature sources report on the effectivity of MTX. However, MTX monotherapy is not always sufficiently effective. In these cases, successful combination therapy with acitretin has been reported, particularly for the pustular forms (9), and the use of TNF-α antagonists also seems to be promising here (10). In addition, studies are investigating the approval of IL-36 antibodies for the treatment of generalized pustular psoriasis, which have shown promising results so far (11).

8.2.3. Methotrexate in combination with other therapeutic agents

8.2.3.1. Combination with external therapeutic agents

Combination with topical corticosteroids

Accompanying topical therapy is usually necessary when treating psoriasis vulgaris. Even if the additional effect of topically applied corticosteroids is only insufficiently documented in clinical studies, daily experience in practice shows their good effectivity. A combination with steroids can achieve a faster therapeutic effect, especially in the initial phase of MTX treatment. Since it can be assumed that topical treatment can be reduced approximately four weeks later if systemic therapy with MTX and local therapy with a corticoid are started concomitantly, the corticoid can be used more generously than would otherwise be recommended in view of its long-term side effects.

Combination with vitamin D3 analogues

There are currently three active ingredients available in Germany for topical therapy with vitamin D3 analogues: calcipotriol, tacalcitol and calcitriol. Clinical studies only support the combination of systemic MTX with topical calcipotriol ointment (e.g. Daivonex® ointment, Psorcutan® ointment). In a controlled study with 98 long-term MTX patients, the additional benefit and safety of topical calcipotriol were tested in comparison to vehicle (12). The experience when titrating the MTX dosage showed that the doses required to suppress skin symptoms were over 3 mg per week lower with simultaneous use of topical calcipotriol-containing ointment compared with simultaneous application of the vehicle, i.e. calcipotriol had an MTX-sparing effect. Furthermore, after discontinuation of MTX, the time until recurrence of skin symptoms and the frequency of recurrences were significantly delayed using topical calcipotriol. The spectrum of side effects remained unchanged with combination therapy compared to the respective monotherapy.

Combination with topical steroids/vitamin D3 analogues as a combination preparation

Currently, in Germany, the fixed combination of betamethasone and calcipotriol is recommended as a topical first-line therapy for both acute and long-term treatment, as it has a better therapeutic effect than the use of the individual substances alone, as well as a low side effect profile. After initially daily application, maintenance therapy twice weekly is recommended where necessary (13).

Clinical studies on the combination with MTX are not available, but experience in practice shows good efficacy, analogous to the use of the individual substances, with the same range of side effects.

Combination with dithranol

There are no controlled clinical studies using this combination, although it is often chosen in clinical practice. In a retrospective study in which dithranol was used as part of the Ingram regimen (tar bath, UV irradiation, dithranol), it was shown that the administration of 15 mg MTX per week from the second or third week of treatment over an average of 29 months could significantly extend the time to relapse (14). The time until the psoriatic lesions healed was five weeks on average. The MTX dose was then gradually reduced after 10 months in patients who were symptom-free. In our own experience, this treatment is similarly effective as dithranol alone, possibly combined with bath PUVA therapy.

Combination with UV therapy

There are several studies that examine the efficacy and safety of a combination of MTX with different qualities of ultraviolet light. However, these are all studies with small patient numbers. In some cases, there is no real control group, so the doses of UV light required alongside MTX are compared with the doses available from the patient's medical history. The most recent study compares the combination of narrowband UVB therapy with MTX versus placebo, with the administration of MTX or placebo being randomized (15). All studies come to the conclusion that the combination of broadband UVB, narrowband UVB or PUVA with MTX offers clear advantages in terms of effectivity. The time to healing or the number of radiation sessions required is significantly reduced when combined with MTX and the time until a recurrence occurs is prolonged.

Critics of the combination therapy of MTX with UV light refer to a possibly increased risk of the development of malignant neoplasms of the skin (16, 17). This risk is seen primarily in combination with systemic PUVA. MTX therapy alone does not appear to lead to an increased incidence of malignant neoplasms of the skin. However, it is unclear whether it promotes the development of such tumors when radiation is used at the same time, for example through an immunosuppressive effect. There are still no good epidemiological studies on this issue.

8.2.3.2. Combinations with systemic therapeutics

Combination with systemic corticosteroids

Although the combination of MTX with systemic corticosteroids is still frequently used in the treatment of psoriatic arthritis, it should be used very cautiously in the treatment of psoriatic skin changes – if at all. This option is no longer mentioned in the current AWMF guideline.

Combination with retinoids

The success of a combination of MTX with acitretin or etretinate in the treatment of severe cases of psoriasis, especially pustular psoriasis, has been described several times in the literature. However, this combination can lead to severe toxic hepatitis, so it should be reserved for exceptional, treatment-resistant cases.

Combination with ciclosporin A

MTX and ciclosporin A (CsA) have been used successfully as a combination in rheumatology for many years. In a case collection of 12 patients who received this treatment for more than 1 year, six developed renal insufficiency, which was not fully reversible in three of these patients. We now have the results of two prospective studies in which the efficacy and safety of the combination were investigated in patients with psoriatic arthritis (PsA) (18) and psoriasis vulgaris (19). Aydin and colleagues (19) applied consistant doses of 10 mg MTX intramuscularly per week in combination with 2.5 mg/kg CsA per day over an average treatment period of 10 weeks. The combination achieved a reduction in the median PASI of 77%. No serious side effects were reported. Fraser and colleagues (18) treated PsA patients with low PASI values; the effectivity of the combination treatment of at least 15 mg MTX per week and 2.5 to 4 mg CsA/kg on the skin is therefore difficult to assess. In this study, more adverse events, including 4 serious ones, were recorded in the MTX/CsA combination group over a treatment period of 12 weeks compared to the MTX/placebo group. 4 patients in the MTX/CsA group had to discontinue the study due to abnormal laboratory values.

Overall, the risks of combination MTX/CsA treatment appear to be significantly higher than for either substance as monotherapy. It is therefore questionable whether this combination is still appropriate, given the large number of biologics and alternative combination options now available.

Combination with biologics

The combination of MTX with the TNF-α inhibitors infliximab, etanercept (ETA), adalimumab, certolizumab pegol and golimumab is established in rheumatology and is currently being expanded with biosimilars. These combinations can be considered well tolerated due to the much lower organ toxicity of the biologicals. The successful use of a combination of TNF-α inhibitors and MTX has also been repeatedly reported in the treatment of psoriasis vulgaris.

Zachariae et al. were able to show in 59 patients with psoriasis that the continuous combined administration of ETA with MTX over 24 weeks was superior to treatment with ETA and a reduction of MTX dosage (20). In recent years, a large number of other biologicals, such as IL-17 and IL-23 inhibitors, have found their way into the treatment of psoriasis vulgaris. Due to the high effectivity of these substance groups, the combination with MTX has become less important for these preparations, in contrast to TNF blockers.

The research is therefore very clear and there are a few studies on the combination of IL-17 antibodies with MTX in PsA and so far no studies on the combination of IL-23 blockers with MTX for dermatological issues.

In an open label study from 2020, the administration of ixekizumab (IXE) (IL-17 antibody) in combination with and without MTX was compared in patients with PsA. To assess the cutaneous effect, the primary endpoint in this study was the PASI 100 response (i.e. the complete absence of skin symptoms) after 52 weeks. Similar results were found in both groups. The primary endpoint was achieved by 63.5% of patients with the combination therapy IXE/MTX and by 65.5% of patients with IXE alone (21).

Unfortunately, a final assessment of the combination of MTX with IL-23 or IL-17 inhibitors cannot be made due to the very limited data available.

Combination with other therapeutic agents

Successful combination treatments of MTX with other systemic therapeutic agents are sporadically reported in the literature. These include fumaric acid esters and colchicine for the treatment of severe and pustular forms of psoriasis. To date, there are only isolated case reports for these combinations.

8.2.4. Psoriasis-specific safety aspects of the use of methotrexate

MTX is a drug with considerable potential for side effects and therefore requires the physician to have comprehensive knowledge of the expected range of side effects and experience in the use of systemic therapies. Adequate patient compliance is also essential.

☞ also Chapter 10.

Detailed recommendations for the use of MTX for psoriasis can be found in the current S3 guideline (22). Therefore, only a few special features of the treatment of psoriasis vulgaris with MTX are mentioned here. The risk of concurrent malignant diseases for psoriasis patients using MTX was investigated in the 1980s in two retrospective studies on large groups (23, 24). In these studies, no increased risk of malignant diseases could be demonstrated. Current data from the PSOLAR (Psoriasis Longitudinal Assessment and Registry), an international registry established in 2007, confirm this. In a case-control analysis of registry data from 12,090 patients, no increased incidence of malignancies (excluding non-melanoma skin cancer (NMSC)) could be found using MTX (both for short-term and long-term use over more than 12 months) (25).

According to the available data, the extent to which MTX increases the risk of NMSC cannot be clearly assessed – in contrast to CsA. For psoriasis, there is one study that indicates a relative risk of 2.0 (93% CI 1.4-2.8) after adjustment for PUVA therapy. However, three other studies found no association (26).

Registry data from PSOLAR, published in 2019, showed an increased risk of basal cell carcinoma after MTX exposure, but the risk of cutaneous squamous cell carcinoma was unchanged (27).

In the past, the induction of liver fibrosis was seen as a dose-dependent complication. More recent data could not confirm this assumption. Therefore, the liver biopsy recommended in the past when a cumulative MTX dose of 1.0-1.5 g was reached is no longer recommended. High-resolution sonography of the liver and, if necessary, the determination of the amino-terminal propeptide

Diagnostics	Time			
	before treatment	within the first 2 weeks	during the first 2 months, once every 4 weeks	then every 3 months
Blood count (including differential blood count)*	✔	✔	✔	✔
Liver enzymes**	✔		✔	✔
Serum creatinine	✔		✔	✔
Urine status	✔			
Pregnancy test (urine or blood)	✔			
Interferon gamma release assay (IGRA) (to rule out tuberculosis)	✔			
Hepatitis B and hepatitis C serology	✔			
HIV serology	✔			
Serum albumin***	✔		✔	✔
Aminoterminal procollagen peptide (PIIINP), if available****	✔		alle 3 Monate	

Table 8.1: Monitoring of psoriasis patients using MTX. According to AWMF Guidelines Register, No.: 013 - 001, 2021 Development stage 3: Treatment of psoriasis vulgaris (22).
* if leukocytes <3.0, neutrophils <1.0, platelets <100, dose reduction or end of therapy.
** if liver values >2-3 ´ higher than baseline values: initiate further diagnostics (repeat determination/consult hepatologist) and consider dose reduction or stop therapy.
*** in selected cases (e.g. if hypoalbuminemia is suspected or in patients taking other medications with a high binding affinity for serum albumin).
****If PIIINP values are abnormal during treatment with MTX, a hepatologist should be consulted.

of type III procollagen in the serum have now been established as non-invasive monitoring procedures.

Currently, the laboratory tests listed in Table 8.1 are recommended for monitoring from a dermatological perspective.

The administration of folic acid 12-24 hours after administration of MTX can reduce the toxicity of MTX in the treatment of RA. There are conflicting data on this for psoriasis. In some cases, a reduction in effectivity due to the administration of folate has been described. However, the current S3 guideline recommends the administration of 5 mg folic acid once a week 24 hours after administration of MTX.

Another long-neglected aspect of psoriasis vulgaris is the increased mortality, particularly due to cardiovascular disease. Gelfand et al., using data from the General Practice Research Database in Great Britain from the period 1988-2003, showed that male and female patients with severe psoriasis died 3.5 years (95% CI 1.2-5.8) and 4.4 years (95% CI 2.2-6.6) earlier, respectively, than the comparison population (28).

A case control analysis of data from the PSOLAR registry showed that systemic therapy for psoriasis can have a positive effect on mortality. At the cut-off point of the analysis in August 2018, 12,090 patients had been observed for a median period of 6.8 years. Treatment with MTX was able to reduce mortality statistically significantly within a treatment period of at least one year (29).

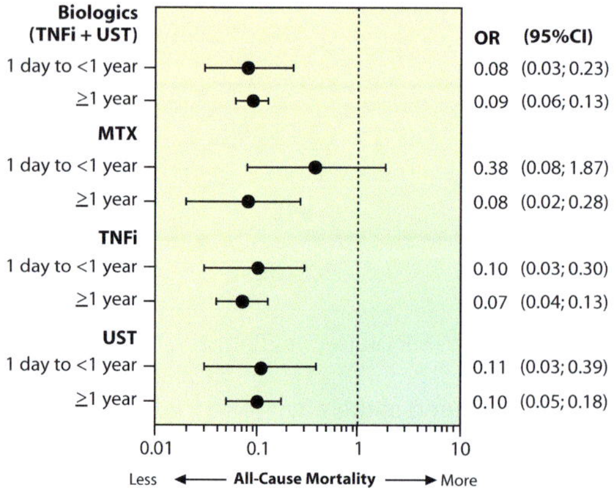

Figure 8.2: Comparison of the change in mortality risk in psoriasis patients with systemic therapy for less than or more than one year (29).

8.3. Methotrexate in the treatment of localized scleroderma

Localized scleroderma (morphea, LSC) is a rare fibrosing disease of the skin which, unlike systemic scleroderma, does not affect any internal organs. The disease is usually self-limiting with a spontaneous remission rate of over 50% within 5 years. However, a subgroup of patients develops pronounced fibrosis and extensive involvement of the integument with sometimes severe signs of inflammation, which can lead to considerable cosmetic distress and the development of contractures. A whole range of therapeutic approaches such as CsA or vitamin D analogues have been described as helpful in case reports and smaller case studies.

There is currently one placebo-controlled multicenter study (30) on the treatment of LSC with MTX, which was able to confirm the observations of the effectivity of MTX in this group of diseases in a number of case series and non-controlled studies. This randomized, double-blind, placebo-controlled study included 70 children with LS (46 patients in the MTX group and 24 in the placebo group). In the MTX group, there was a significant improvement in skin involvement compared to placebo. The rate of recurrences was also significantly lower after MTX therapy (33%) compared to placebo (71%) (30). Since different dosages for MTX and glucocorticosteroids were used in the studies mentioned above, CARRA (Childhood Arthritis and Rheumatology Research Alliance) created three different "therapy pathways" for the treatment of LS in childhood for the first time in 2012: MTX monotherapy, MTX steroid pulse therapy with intravenous methylprednisolone, and MTX steroid pulse therapy with MTX and oral prednisone (31). Treatment of LS is recommended in patients with severe skin involvement and/or musculoskeletal involvement. The duration of treatment should be at least 12 months. A detailed treatment algorithm using MTX for LS can be found in the updated S2-K guideline (AWMF register no.: 013/66).

8.4. Methotrexate in the treatment of bullous dermatoses

8.4.1. Bullous pemphigoid and related diseases

Bullous pemphigoid primarily affects older patients over 65 years of age and has a high mortality rate if left untreated. According to newer pathophysiological concepts, mucous membrane pemphigoid, herpes gestationis and linear IgA dermatosis are also included in this group of diseases. If the integument is severely involved, systemic treatment with corticosteroids is usually essential. The dosage is usually 0.5 to 1.0 mg/kg per day prednisone equivalent. However, the use of higher steroid doses in this patient group is associated with increased mortality. Therefore, MTX was started early on as a steroid-sparing immunosuppressant in the treatment of bullous pemphigoid. However, the first large non-controlled study was not published until 1994 by Paul et al. (32).

For bullous pemphigoid, there is also a non-controlled study in which patients (<70 years) with pemphigoid disease that could not be controlled by topical steroids were treated with MTX monotherapy (5-12.5 mg per week orally). This approach led to complete remission in 7 of the 11 patients treated (33). These results are supported by a study by Dereure et al., who investigated MTX as a systemic "mono"therapy in addition to the use of topical steroids. They were able to achieve remission in 17/18 patients with doses between 7.5 and 15 mg per day. Similar results with a response rate of 70-90% were also reported for the treatment of ocular cicatricial pemphigoid (34).

MTX continues to be part of the list of medications recommended for cortisone-sparing immunosuppressive therapy of moderate to severe bullous pemphigoid in the current AWMF guideline (S2-K Register No. 013-071;).

8.4.2. Pemphigus vulgaris

The successful use of MTX in the treatment of pemphigus vulgaris was first reported in 1969 by Peck and Ossermann (35). Since then, over 12 studies have been published describing the use of MTX in patients with pemphigus vulgaris. These studies were not conducted double-blind. Nevertheless, with over 153 published patients, MTX is one of the best-documented immunosuppressants in the treatment of pemphigus vulgaris after azathioprine. In these studies, MTX was introduced into therapy as a corticosteroid-sparing drug (which is initially used in doses of 2-3 mg/kg per day for this disease). Most studies used doses between 10 and 30 mg per week via different application routes. A response was usually observed within 2-4 weeks, so that the concomitant steroid medication could then be reduced as much as possible. Due to the significantly greater disease activity of pemphigus vulgaris in many patients compared to bullous pemphigoid, MTX, like the drugs azathioprine or mycofenolat mofetil, which are comparable in terms of effectivity, is not sufficiently effective in all patients. In this case, alternative therapeutic approaches such as immunoadsorption, immunoglobulins and, more recently, CD20 antibodies such as rituximab come into consideration, which can then also be used in combination with MTX. Here, too, reference is made to the recently updated AWMF guideline (S2-K Register No. 013-071;).

8.5. Methotrexate in the treatment of atopic dermatitis

Atopic eczema is a chronic, inflammatory skin disease that affects children and adults. Systemic immunomodulatory treatment is an option for patients in whom topical treatment, including potent corticosteroids, also in combination with light therapy, is not able to adequately control the disease. The dosages described in case reports and case series for the use of MTX in atopic eczema correspond to the dosages for other chronic inflammatory diseases. In a single-blind study (36), the use of MTX at a dosage of 10-22.5 mg per week was compared with the use of azathioprine at a dosage of 1.5-2.5 mg/kg per day over a period of 24 weeks. After 12 weeks of treatment, both patient groups had a comparable significant improvement of approximately 40%. The side effect profile was comparable for both drugs. However, with the introduction of effective biologics with few side effects such as dupilumab and tralokinumab, as well as the recent approval of JAK inhibitors such as baricitinib, upadacitinib and abrocitinib, MTX can now only be seen as a reserve medication in the treatment of severe atopic eczema (37).

8.6. Methotrexate for the treatment of rare skin diseases

In a number of rare or very rare skin diseases, MTX can be considered as a therapeutic option based on a number of positive case reports or case series. These include chronic inflammatory diseases such as cutaneous sarcoidosis, pityriasis rubra pilaris and orofacial granulomatosis (cheilitis granulomatosa). In the treatment of mycosis fungoides, MTX is part of the current guideline recommendations for stages Ib - IIb.

8.7. References

1. Genestier L, Paillot R, Quemeneur L, Izeradjene K, and Revillard JP. Mechanisms of action of methotrexate. Immunopharmacology 2000;47:247-257.

2. Weinstein GD, Jeffes E, McCullough JL. Cytotoxic and immunologic effects of methotrexate in psoriasis. J Invest Dermatol 1990;95:49S-52S.

3. Chan ES, Cronstein BN. Molecular action of methotrexate in inflammatory diseases. Arthritis Res 2002;4: 266-273.

4. Weinstein GD, Frost P. Methotrexate for psoriasis. A new therapeutic schedule. Arch Dermatol 1971;103:33-38.

5. Collins P, Rogers S. The efficacy of methotrexate in psoriasis—a review of 40 cases. Clin Exp Dermatol 1992; 17:257-260

6. Spuls PI, Witkamp L, Bossuyt PM, Bos JD. Asystematic review of five systemic treatments for severe psoriasis. Br J Dermatol 1997;137:943-949.

7. Warren RB, Mrowietz U, von Kiedrowski R, Niesmann J, Wilsmann-Theis D, Ghoreschi K, Zschocke I, Falk TM, Blödorn-Schlicht N, Reich K. An intensified dosing schedule of subcutaneous methotrexate in patients with moderate to severe plaque-type psoriasis (METOP): a 52 week, multicentre, randomised, double-blind, placebo-controlled, phase 3 trial. Lancet 2017;389: 528-537.

8. Reich K, Sorbe C, Griese L, Reich JLK, Augustin M. The value of subcutaneous vs. oral methotrexate: real-world data from the German psoriasis registry Pso Best. Br J Dermatol 2021;184:765-767.

9. Tuyp E, MacKie RM. Combination therapy for psoriasis with methotrexate and etretinate. J Am Acad Dermatol 1986; 14:70-73.

10. Viguier M, Aubin F, Delaporte E, Pagès C, Paul C, Beylot-Barry M, Gouhon C, Rybojad M, Bachelez H, Groupe de Recherche sur le Psoriasis de la SociétéFrancaise de Dermatologie. Efficacy and safety of tumor necrosis factor inhibitors in acute generalized pustular psoriasis. Arch Dermatol 2012;148: 1423-1425.

11. Bachelez H, Choon SE, Marrakchi S, Burden AD, Tsai TF, Morita A, Navarini AA, Zheng M, Xu J, Turki H, Anadkat MJ, Rajeswari S, Hua H, Vulcu SD, Hall D, Tetzlaff K, Thoma C, Lebwohl MG; Effisayil. Trial Investigators. Trial of spesolimab for generalized pustular psoriasis. N Engl J Med 2021;385: 2431-2440.

12. de Jong EM, Mork NJ, Seijger MM, De La Brassine M, Lauharanta J, Jansen CT, Guilhou JJ, Guillot B, Ostrojic A, Souteyrand P, et al. The combination of calcipotriol and methotrexate compared with methotrexate and vehicle in psoriasis: results of a 101 multicentre placebo-controlled randomized trial. Br J Dermatol 2003;148: 318-325.

13. Körber A, Wilsmann-Theis D, Augustin M, von Kiedrowski R, Mrowietz U, Rosenbach T, Meller S, Pinter A, Sticherling M, Gerdes S; PsoNetFörderverein. Topische Therapie bei Psoriasis vulgaris – ein Behandlungspfad. J Dtsch Dermatol Ges Suppl 2019;4:3-14

14. van de Kerkhof PC, Mali JW. Methotrexate maintenance following Ingram therapy in 'difficult' psoriasis. Br J Dermatol 1982;106:623-627.

15. Asawanonda P, Nateetongrungsak Y. Methotrexate plus narrowband UVB phototherapy versus narrowband UVB phototherapy alone in the treatment of plaque-type psoriasis: a randomized, placebocontrolled study. J Am Acad Dermatol 2006;54:1013-1018.

16. MacKie RM, Fitzsimons CP. Risk of carcinogenicity in patients with psoriasis treated with methotrexate or PUVA singly or in combination. J Am Acad Dermatol 1983;9:467-469.

17. Fitzsimons CP, Long J, MacKie RM. Synergistic carcinogenic potential of methotrexate and PUVA in psoriasis. Lancet 1983;1:235-236.

18. Fraser AD, Kuijk AW, Westhovens R, Karim Z, Wakefield R, Gerards AH, Landewe R, Steinfeld SD, Emery P, Dijkmans BA, et al. A randomised, double blind, placebo controlled, multicenter trial of combination therapy with methotrexate plus ciclosporin in patients with active psoriatic arthritis. Ann Rheum Dis 2005;64:859-864.

19. Aydin F, Canturk T, Senturk N, Turanli AY. Methotrexate and ciclosporin combination for the treatment of severe psoriasis. Clin Exp Dermatol 2006;31:520-524.

20. Zachariae C, Mork NJ, Reunala T, Lorentzen H, Falk E, Karvonen SL, Johannesson A, Clareus B, Skov L, Mork G, Walker S, Qvitzau S. The combination of etanercept and methotrexate increases the effectiviness of treatment in active psoriasis despite inadequate effect of methotrexate therapy. Acta DermVenerol 2008;88:495-501.

21. Smolen JS, Sebba A, Ruderman EM, Schulze-Koops H, Sapin C, Gellett AM, Sprabery AT, Li L, de la Torre I, Gallo G, Liu-Leage S, Pillai S, Reis P, Nash P 2020. Efficacy and safety of ixekizumab with or without methotrexate in biologic-naïve patients with psoriatic arthritis: 52-week results from SPIRIT-H2H Study. RheumatolTher. 7:1021-1035

22. "Therapie der Psoriasis vulgaris" (AWMF Leitlinien Register Nr. 013/001,2021, Entwicklungsstufe 3, http://www.uni-duesseldorf.de/AWMF/ll/013-001.htm).

23. Nyfors A, Jensen H. Frequency of malignant neoplasms in 248 long-term methotrexate-treated psoriatics. A preliminary study. Dermatologica 1983;167:260-261.

24. Stern RS, Zierler S, Parrish JA. Methotrexate used for psoriasis and the risk of noncutaneous or cutaneous malignancy. Cancer 1982;50:869-872.

25. Fiorentino D, Ho V, Lebwohl MG, Leite L, Hopkins L, Galindo C, Goyal K, Langholff W, Fakharzadeh S, Srivastava B, Langley RG. Risk of malignancy with systemic psoriasis treat-

ment in the Psoriasis Longitudinal Assessment Registry. J Am Acad Dermatol 2017;77:845-854.

26. Krathen MS, Gottlieb AB, Mease PJ. Pharmacologic immunodulation and cutaneous malignancy in rheumatoid arthritis, psoriasis and psoriatic arthritis. J Rheumatol 2010;37: 2205-2215.

27. deShazo R, Soltani-Arabshahi R, Krishnasamy S, Langley RG, Kalia S, Ståhle M, Langholff W, Goyal K, Fakharzadeh S, Galindo C, Srivastava B, Krueger G. Non-melanoma skin cancer risk among patients in the Psoriasis Longitudinal Assessment and Registry (PSOLAR). J Drugs Dermatol 2019;18: 1059-1060.

28. Gelfand JM, Troxel AB, Lewis JD, Kurd SK, Shin DB, Wang X, Margolis DJ, Strom BL. The risk of mortality in patients with psoriasis: results from a population-based study. Arch Dermatol 2007;143:1493-9.

29. Langley RG, Poulin Y, Srivastava B, Lafferty KP, Fakharzadeh S, Langholff W, Augustin M. Reduced risk of mortality associated with systemic psoriasis treatment in the Psoriasis Longitudinal Assessment and Registry (PSOLAR): A nested case-control analysis. J Am Acad Dermatol 2021;84:60-69.

30. Zulian F, Martini G, Vallongo C, Vittadello F, Falcini F, Patrizi A, Alessio M, La Torre F, Podda RA, Gerloni V, Cutrone M, Belloni-Fortina A, Paradisi M, Martino S, Perilongo G. Methotrexate treatment in juvenile localized scleroderma: a randomized, double-blind, placebo-controlled trial. Arthritis Rheum 2011;63:1998-2006.

31. Li SC, Torok KS, Pope E, et al. Development of consensus treatment plans for juvenile localized scleroderma: a roadmap toward comparative effectiveness studies in juvenile localized scleroderma. Arthritis Care Res (Hoboken) 2012;64:1175-1185.

32. Paul MA, Jorizzo JL, Fleischer AB Jr, White WL. Low-dose methotrexate treatment in elderly patients with bullous pemphigoid. J Am Acad Dermatol 1994;31:620-625.

33. Heilborn JD, Stahle-Backdahl M, Albertioni F, Vassilaki I, Peterson C, Stephansson E. Low-dose oral pulse methotrexate as monotherapy in elderly patients with bullous pemphigoid. J Am Acad Dermatol 1999;40:741-749.

34. McCluskey P, Chang JH, Singh R, Wakefield D. Methotrexate therapy for ocular cicatricial pemphigoid. Ophthalmology 2004;111:796-801.

35. Peck SM, Osserman KE. Studies in bullous diseases: treatment of pemphigus vulgaris with methotrexate, two patients (one with concurrent myasthenia gravis). J Mt Sinai Hosp N Y 1969;36:71-76.

36. Schram ME, Roekevisch E, Leeflang MMG, Bos JD, Schmitt J, Spuls Pl. A randomized trial of methotrexate versus azathioprine for severe atopic eczema. J Allergy Clin Immunol 2011;128:353-359.

37. Choyativa R, Paler A. JAK inhibitors in the treatment of atopic dermatitis. J Allergy Clin Immunol 2021; 148(4):927-940.

9. Methotrexate in gastroenterology

The use of methotrexate (MTX) for various rheumatic diseases has a long history. MTX has not yet achieved such decisive importance in gastroenterological diseases, although it has been scientifically investigated and used for various gastroenterological diseases for more than 25 years. Most studies using MTX in gastroenterology were carried out on patients with chronic inflammatory bowel disease and the study results were partly inconsistent. Despite many positive study results for Crohn's disease, the use of MTX for this indication is rather infrequent. In the following chapter, the data supporting the use of MTX in various gastroenterological diseases are presented and the possible inclusion of MTX into treatment algorithms is discussed.

9.1. Methotrexate for Crohn's disease

The use of MTX for Crohn's disease focuses primarily on patients with steroid-dependent Crohn's disease. To avoid side effects of long-term cortisone therapy, current German and international guidelines recommend the use of immunosuppressants or biologics. Although thiopurines have historically and quantitatively accounted for the largest proportion used for this purpose, MTX is a highly effective and well-researched immunosuppressive substance that can reduce steroid use in these patients. In a large randomized study, which historically represents a "landmark study", the use of MTX in 141 patients at a dosage of 25 mg per week intramuscularly was investigated (1). In the MTX group, 39% of patients were able to achieve remission compared to 19% in the placebo group ($p=0.025$; Number Needed To Treat, NNT=5). In addition, there is study experience in other smaller populations. With regard to induction of remission in Crohn's disease, a total of seven randomized controlled trials were examined in a Cochrane analysis (2). The meta-analysis concluded that intramuscular injection of MTX at 25 mg per week shows a benefit in terms of remission induction and the achievement of steroid-free remission. Lower oral doses do not appear to have a sufficient effect in remission induction, although the available studies are small and probably not sufficiently conclusive. Comparative studies between MTX and other immunosuppressants such as azathioprine (AZA) or 6-mercaptopurine in patients with steroid-dependent Crohn's disease showed no significant differences between the two substance groups, neither in terms of remission induction nor remission maintenance (3, 4). In a network meta-analysis, no significant differences were found between MTX and AZA with regard to remission induction and remission maintenance (5). In terms of side effects, no differences were found between MTX and thiopurines in the majority of the admittedly relatively small studies.

Since the combination therapy of infliximab (INX) with AZA showed a therapeutic benefit in both remission induction and remission maintenance in patients with Crohn's disease (6) as well as ulcerative colitis (7), it was investigated whether a combination of MTX with INX had an additional benefit compared to INX monotherapy. In this study, no significant effect on remission induction was found in patients who were treated with MTX in addition to INX (8). However, with regard to the formation of autoantibodies against INX, a preventive effect was found in the combination therapy with a significant reduction in autoantibody formation from 20% when using INX monotherapy to 4% when using combination therapy (9). Data on combination therapies with MTX and ustekinumab (UST) or vedolizumab (VDZ) are not available.

MTX also has a proven role in maintaining remission in patients with Crohn's disease as monotherapy. In the previously described "landmark study" of steroid-dependent Crohn's disease patients, patients who had been treated with 25 mg MTX intramuscularly per week for 16 weeks were continued on a maintenance regime of 15 mg MTX intramuscularly per week and compared to placebo. 61% of patients who were treated with MTX for a further 40 weeks showed remission after this period compared to 39% in the placebo group ($p<0.04$, NNT=4) (10). A Cochrane meta-analysis on the value of MTX for maintaining remission in Crohn's disease concluded that the benefit of parenteral MTX treatment at a dose of at least

15 mg is reasonable and should be preferred to oral treatment and lower doses.

Based on the study data, MTX has also been assigned a role in remission maintenance therapy for Crohn's disease in national and European guidelines (11, 12). However, due to the significantly fewer data available compared to thiopurines, remission maintenance with MTX is generally only considered if thiopurines are not tolerated or are ineffective (11).

There are conflicting data regarding the rate of mucosal healing using MTX in patients with Crohn's disease. While the study by Lahari described only 11% mucosal healing rates using MTX compared to AZA (50%) or INX (60%), another study by Manosa showed 40-50% mucosal healing in Crohn's disease patients.

In small studies, MTX has also shown some effectivity in the treatment of fistulizing Crohn's disease, and complete fistula closure has been documented in 22-50% of patients (13).

Due to its excellent efficacy and many years of experience in rheumatology, MTX is also often recommended for joint-related extraintestinal manifestations of Crohn's disease, particularly in severe peripheral arthritis.

There are only a few studies investigating the application route of MTX in Crohn's disease. Since MTX is absorbed in the proximal jejunum, the absorption and bioavailability of MTX can be reduced, especially in patients with small intestinal involvement. In patients with Crohn's disease who are in remission, two studies have shown a bioavailability of 73-86% for the oral route compared to subcutaneous application (14, 15). Since it is well documented that subcutaneous administration is superior to oral administration in patients with RA, parenteral administration is preferred to oral administration in Crohn's disease. Ready-to-use syringes for subcutaneous injection of MTX are available in Germany and the drug is approved for the treatment of mild to moderate Crohn's disease alone or in combination with corticosteroids in adults who do not respond to or cannot tolerate thiopurines.

In a large retrospective study, the effectivity of MTX was also demonstrated in pediatric patients with Crohn's disease. This study showed only a slight advantage of the parenteral route over the oral route of administration (16).

There is no reliable data regarding the duration of MTX use. According to expert opinion, a treatment duration of at least 12-16 months is required, possibly even longer (17).

Based on current study data, the national DGVS guidelines consider the use of MTX in patients with steroid-dependent Crohn's disease equivalent to other immunosuppressants, biologics and small molecules (11) (☞ Figure 9.1). In clinical practice, however, MTX is rarely used as a primary treatment option for this indication, but rather in cases of thiopurine-refractory disease, thiopurine intolerance or the simultaneous occurrence of extraintestinal manifestations with joint involvement. However, the data on the use of MTX in extraintestinal manifestations is also rather limited and the indication is more likely to be extrapolated based on promising data from rheumatology.

The use of MTX is also recommended in the European ECCO guidelines, but only in the maintenance of remission and in the treatment of steroid-dependent Crohn's disease when other medications are not available (12). MTX is also used in pediatrics based on a number of retrospective cohort studies. Recommendations are available for its use in the maintenance of steroid-free remission in young patients with severe disease and poor prognosis (18).

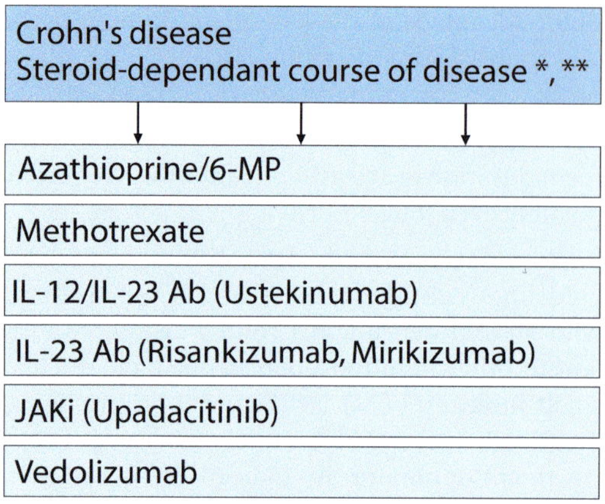

Figure 9.1: Use of MTX in steroid-dependent Crohn's disease. MTX is recommended in the national guidelines as a treatment option for both remission induction and remission maintenance in steroid-dependent Crohn's disease. The DGVS guideline recommends MTX for this indication on an equal footing with thiopurines, TNF antibodies, JAK inhibitors, IL-12/IL-23 antibodies, IL-23 antibodies and vedolizumab. The treatment decision for one or the other immunosuppressant is individualized. The European guidelines also do not prioritize any of the various treatment options for this indication, but give MTX a rather subordinate role due to the limited data available.
* The drugs are listed alphabetically. This order does not imply prioritization for clinical use.
** Alternative depending on the pattern of involvement: surgery.

9.2. Methotrexate for ulcerative colitis

The use of MTX in patients with ulcerative colitis is much more controversial than in patients with Crohn's disease, and there is less evidence for its effectivity. Various case series have shown that MTX effects in ulcerative colitis are similar to those in Crohn's disease when given parenterally (subcutaneously or intramuscularly) at a dose of 25 mg per week, analogous to the Crohn's disease study (19). However, a prospective controlled study in steroid-dependent ulcerative colitis showed no significant differences in terms of clinical remission between the administration of oral MTX at a dose of 12.5 mg per week compared to placebo (20). However, in this study, a comparatively low dose of MTX was used via oral route. Another prospectively randomized and double-blinded study on the use of MTX in steroid-dependent ulcerative colitis (METEOR study) compared parenteral administration of MTX at a dose of 25 mg per week (subcutaneously or intramuscularly) with placebo in 111 patients with ulcerative colitis, but failed to meet the primary endpoint of the study (21). However, the proportion of patients in steroid-free clinical remission at week 16 was significantly higher in the MTX group at 42% of patients compared to 24% in the placebo group (p=0.04). A Cochrane analysis on the role of MTX in the induction of remission in patients with ulcerative colitis, which did not include this study, shows no significant effect in terms of remission induction in patients with ulcerative colitis receiving MTX compared to the placebo group (22). Another Cochrane meta-analysis also failed to demonstrate a significant effect of MTX in maintaining remission (23). The MERIT-UC study investigated the effectivity of MTX for maintaining remission in ulcerative colitis (24). 91 patients (51%) achieved a clinical response in week 16, of which 84 patients were included in the maintenance study. In week 48, 30% of the patients in the placebo group (12/40) and 27% of the patients in the MTX group (12/44) were in steroid-free remission (p=0.86). There was also no significant effect in the other subgroups that would justify remission-maintenance therapy with MTX in ulcerative colitis. At the present time, MTX is therefore not recommended for remission induction and remission maintenance in ulcerative colitis based on the existing data in national and international guidelines.

9.3. Mechanism of action of methotrexate in chronic inflammatory bowel disease

MTX's mechanism of action for immunosuppression in chronic inflammatory bowel disease is not fully understood. However, it is probably not significantly different than in other chronic inflammatory diseases and is largely based on inhibition of JAK/STAT signal transduction (25, 26). It was recently shown that the composition of genes in the gut microbiome that are involved in the metabolism of MTX differs between MTX responders and non-responders in RA (27). Similar changes in the gut microbiome could also be present in other chronic inflammatory diseases and may explain differences in the clinical efficacy of MTX in chronic inflammatory bowel disease.

9.4. Side effects of methotrexate therapy for gastrointestinal diseases

The side effects of parenteral or oral MTX therapy do not differ significantly from the side effects in other indications. Common side effects are nausea and anorexia or occasionally stomatitis or diarrhea. More serious side effects include potential hepatotoxicity, bone marrow toxicity (28) and, rarely, hypersensitivity pneumonitis and opportunistic infections (29). An increased risk of lymphomas or neoplasia has not yet been described in long-term MTX therapy (30). In the ECCO guidelines, MTX was therefore classified as relatively safe with regard to the development of malignancy and also when used in patients with previous neoplasia (31).

A particular concern focuses on the development of liver fibrosis or cirrhosis. The feared risk of this side effect relates primarily to a study in which a high incidence of liver fibrosis and cirrhosis was described in patients with psoriasis using MTX (32). Various studies in patients with chronic inflammatory bowel disease who received a cumulative dose of MTX up to 2.5 g showed an increased rate of liver fibrosis or cirrhosis in the biopsies performed (33, 34). A more common occurrence is probably the short-term increase in transaminases using higher-dose MTX, which was observed in the induction study with 25 mg MTX per week. In the long-term maintenance study with 15 mg MTX, no relevant liver toxicity was observed. In a meta-analysis of the hepatotoxicity of MTX, no relevant differences were found between MTX, thiopurines and placebo (35).

9.5. Risk management when using methotrexate for chronic inflammatory bowel disease

The use of MTX should be accompanied by a careful risk–benefit assessment and detailed patient information. Adequate information also includes detailed instructions on the appropriate injection technique for parenteral administration. To reduce side effects and to better monitor tolerability, most users recommend a gradual increase in dosage up to the effective induction dose of 25 mg. A dose reduction to 15 mg as maintenance therapy should be considered after 16 weeks. Oral administration of 5 mg folic acid on the day after MTX administration is mandatory. MTX use should be avoided in patients with alcohol abuse, obesity, diabetes mellitus, hepatic steatosis and other liver diseases as well as in patients with COPD and other lung diseases. In cases of renal insufficiency, the dose must be adjusted to the renal function. Inter-

Examination parameters	Initial examination	Month 1-6	Month 7 and beyond
Complete blood count including platelets and differential blood count	++	At least monthly*	At least quarterly*
Liver panel: γ-GT (GGT), ALAT (GPT), ASAT (GOT), alkaline phosphatase (AP), albumin, bilirubin	++	At least monthly*	At least quarterly*
Kidney function test: serum creatinine, creatinine clearance if necessary	++	At least monthly*	At least quarterly*
Urine analysis	+	At least monthly*	At least quarterly*
Exclusion of pregnancy	++		
Chest X-ray	++		
Pulmonary function test if necessary	+		
Exclusion of TB, hepatitis B, HIV	+		

Table 9.1: Follow-up examinations when using MTX for chronic inflammatory bowel disease. The initial laboratory tests should be carried out every 7 days in the first 4 weeks, 14-day checks in the second and third month, then at least 4-week intervals are recommended ().

actions with other medications should be considered. Standard infection management, including checking the vaccination status, is no different from other immunosuppressive therapies (36).

According to the recommendation of the Competence Network for Intestinal Diseases, laboratory tests including blood count, liver and kidney panels should be performed weekly for the first 7 days, every 14 days in the second and third months and then at 4-week intervals (☞ Table 9.1).

The contraindications should be taken into account, particularly when considering family planning. Pregnancy has to be ruled out before starting treatment with MTX. If a patient wishes to have children, it should be noted that, according to the recommendations of the German Society for Rheumatology, MTX is strictly contraindicated during pregnancy and breastfeeding and MTX should be discontinued at least three months before conception in both women and men undergoing treatment. When taking MTX during childbearing and fertile age, reliable contraception is absolutely necessary. It should also be noted that after discontinuation, permanent folic acid substitution is required until the end of the pregnancy (37).

9.6. Methotrexate for other gastroenterological diseases

There are only small case reports on the use of MTX for other gastroenterological diseases outside of chronic inflammatory bowel disease. For example, the use of MTX is occasionally recommended for patients with refractory autoimmune hepatitis (38, 39). However, MTX is not approved for the treatment of autoimmune hepatitis.

9.7. Summary

The study data demonstrate a positive effect of MTX in terms of remission induction and remission maintenance in steroid-dependent Crohn's disease, which is also reflected in the recommendations of the national and European guidelines. The use of MTX in patients with ulcerative colitis currently plays no relevant role due to the recent negative study data and also taking into account the increasing number of treatment alternatives.

The rate of side effects of MTX is manageable when used carefully, so there is a good cost–benefit ratio when taking into account the relatively low costs. Nevertheless, the use of MTX currently plays a rather minor role in gastroenterological diseases and the current use in chronic inflammatory bowel diseases is relatively infrequent. However, the effectivity and tolerability of the drug in Crohn's disease are well documented, so there are many arguments in favor of its use for this indication in patients who require immunosuppressive therapy.

In other gastroenterological diseases such as autoimmune hepatitis, MTX is occasionally used as a last resort medication.

9.8. References

1. Feagan BG, Rochon J, Fedorak RN, et al. Methotrexate for the treatment of Crohn's disease. The North American Crohn's Study Group Investigators. N Engl J Med 1995;332: 292-7.

2. McDonald JW, Wang Y, Tsoulis DJ, et al. Methotrexate for induction of remission in refractory Crohn's disease. Cochrane Database Syst Rev 2014;8:CD003459.

3. Patel V, Macdonald JK, McDonald JW, et al. Methotrexate for maintenance of remission in Crohn's disease. Cochrane Database Syst Rev 2009:CD006884.

4. Prefontaine E, Macdonald JK, Sutherland LR. Azathioprine or 6-mercaptopurine for induction of remission in Crohn's disease. Cochrane Database Syst Rev 2010:CD000545.

5. Hazlewood GS, Rezaie A, Borman M, et al. Comparative effectiveness of immunosuppressants and biologics for inducing and maintaining remission in Crohn's disease: a network meta-analysis. Gastroenterology 2015; 148:344-54 e5; quiz e14-5.

6. Colombel JF, Sandborn WJ, Reinisch W, et al. Infliximab, azathioprine, or combination therapy for Crohn's disease. N Engl J Med 2010;362:1383-95.

7. Panaccione R, Ghosh S, Middleton S, et al. Combination therapy with infliximab and azathioprine is superior to monotherapy with either agent in ulcerative colitis. Gastroenterology 2014;146:392-400 e3.

8. Feagan BG, McDonald JW, Panaccione R, et al. Methotrexate in combination with infliximab is no more effective than infliximab alone in patients with Crohn's disease. Gastroenterology 2014;146:681-688 e1.

9. Feagan BG, McDonald JW, Panaccione R, et al. Methotrexate for the prevention of antibodies to infliximab in patients with Crohn's disease. Gastroenterology 2010; A1051.

10. Feagan BG, Fedorak RN, Irvine EJ, et al. A comparison of methotrexate with placebo for the maintenance of remission in Crohn's disease. North American Crohn's Study Group Investigators. N Engl J Med 2000;342:1627-32.

11. Sturm A, Atreya R, Bettenworth D, et al. Aktualisierte S3-Leitlinie "Diagnostik und Therapie des Morbus Crohn" der Deutschen Gesellschaft für Gastroenterologie, Verdauungs- und Stoffwechselkrankheiten (DGVS) Z Gastroenterol 2022; 60:332-418.

12. Torres J, Bonovas S, Doherty G, et al. ECCO Guidelines on Therapeutics in Crohn's Disease: Medical Treatment. J Crohns Colitis 2020;14:4-22.

13. Cassinotti A, Batticciotto A, Parravicini M, et al. Evidence-based efficacy of methotrexate in adult Crohn's disease in different intestinal and extraintestinal indications. Therap Adv Gastroenterol 2022;15:17562848221 085889.

14. Kurnik D, Loebstein R, Fishbein E, et al. Bioavailability of oral vs. subcutaneous low-dose methotrexate in patients with Crohn's disease. Aliment Pharmacol Ther 2003;18:57-63.

15. Wilson A, Patel V, Chande N, et al. Pharmacokinetic profiles for oral and subcutaneous methotrexate in patients with Crohn's disease. Aliment Pharmacol Ther 2013;37:340-5.

16. Turner D, Doveh E, Cohen A, et al. Efficacy of oral methotrexate in paediatric Crohn's disease: a multicentre propensity score study. Gut 2015;64:1898-904.

17. Pittet V, Froehlich F, Maillard MH, et al. When do we dare to stop biological or immunomodulatory therapy for Crohn's disease? Results of a multidisciplinary European expert panel. J Crohns Colitis 2013;7:820-6.

18. Ruemmele FM, Veres G, Kolho KL, et al. Consensus guidelines of ECCO/ESPGHAN on the medical management of pediatric Crohn's disease. J Crohns Colitis 2014; 8:1179-207.

19. Herfarth HH, Osterman MT, Isaacs KL, et al. Efficacy of methotrexate in ulcerative colitis: failure or promise. Inflamm Bowel Dis 2010;16:1421-30.

20. Oren R, Arber N, Odes S, et al. Methotrexate in chronic active ulcerative colitis: a double-blind, randomized, Israeli multicenter trial. Gastroenterology 1996;110: 1416-21.

21. Carbonnel F, Carbonne JF, Filippi J, et al. Methotrexate is not superior to placebo for inducing steroid-free remission, but induces steroid-free clinical remission in a larger proportion of patients with ulcerative colitis. Gastroenterology 2015.

22. Chande N, Wang Y, MacDonald JK, et al. Methotrexate for induction of remission in ulcerative colitis. Cochrane Database Syst Rev 2014;8:CD006618.

23. Wang Y, MacDonald JK, Vandermeer B, et al. Methotrexate for maintenance of remission in ulcerative colitis. Cochrane Database Syst Rev 2015;8:CD007560.

24. Herfarth H, Barnes EL, Valentine JF, et al. Methotrexate is not superior to placebo in maintaining steroid-free response or remission in ulcerative colitis. Gastroenterology 2018;155: 1098-1108 e9.

25. Thomas S, Fisher KH, Snowden JA, et al. Methotrexate is a JAK/STAT pathway inhibitor. PLoS One 2015;10: e0130078.

26. Alqarni AM, Zeidler MP. How does methotrexate work? Biochem Soc Trans 2020;48:559-567.

27. Han M, Zhang N, Mao Y, et al. The potential of gut microbiota metabolic capability to detect drug response in rheumatoid arthritis patients. Front Microbiol 2022; 13:839015.

28. Stein RB, Hanauer SB. Comparative tolerability of treatments for inflammatory bowel disease. Drug Saf 2000;23:429-48.

29. Searles G, McKendry RJ. Methotrexate pneumonitis in rheumatoid arthritis: potential risk factors. Four case reports and a review of the literature. J Rheumatol 1987; 14:1164-71.

30. Salliot C, van der Heijde D. Long-term safety of methotrexate monotherapy in patients with rheumatoid arthritis: a systematic literature research. Ann Rheum Dis 2009;68:1100-4.

31. Annese V, Beaugerie L, Egan L, et al. European evidence-based consensus: Inflammatory bowel disease and malignancies. J Crohns Colitis 2015;9:945-65.

32. Kalb RE, Strober B, Weinstein G, et al. Methotrexate and psoriasis: 2009 National Psoriasis Foundation Consensus Conference. J Am Acad Dermatol 2009;60:824-37.

33. Lemann M, Zenjari T, Bouhnik Y, et al. Methotrexate in Crohn's disease: long-term efficacy and toxicity. Am J Gastroenterol 2000;95:1730-4.

34. Fournier MR, Klein J, Minuk GY, et al. Changes in liver biochemistry during methotrexate use for inflammatory bowel disease. Am J Gastroenterol 2010;105:1620-6.

35. Khan N, Abbas AM, Whang N, et al. Incidence of liver toxicity in inflammatory bowel disease patients treated with methotrexate: a meta-analysis of clinical trials. Inflamm Bowel Dis 2012;18:359-67.

36. Kucharzik T, Ellul P, Greuter T, et al. ECCO Guidelines on the Prevention, Diagnosis, and Management of Infections in Inflammatory Bowel Disease. J Crohns Colitis 2021;15:879-913.

37. Krüger K, Gromnica-Ihle E. Im Auftrag der Kommission für Pharmakotherapie der DGRh. Z Rheumatol 2009;68:169-73.

38. Burak KW, Urbanski SJ, Swain MG. Successful treatment of refractory type 1 autoimmune hepatitis with methotrexate. J Hepatol 1998;29:990-3.

39. Casal Moura M, Liberal R, Cardoso H, et al. Management of autoimmune hepatitis: Focus on pharmacologic treatments beyond corticosteroids. World J Hepatol 2014;6:410-8.

10. Side effects of methotrexate

Methotrexate (MTX), used as chemotherapy of malignant tumors, can cause significant side effects, including mucositis and toxic liver and bone marrow damage (30). Therefore, the use of MTX in the treatment of rheumatism was initially approached with caution. However, increased experience with MTX has led to the abandonment of originally recommended precautions for MTX therapy. These included starting with a reduced dosage (e.g. 7.5 mg per week) and stopping therapy when a certain cumulative dose was reached.

10.1. Toxicity of methotrexate compared to other standard therapeutic agents

MTX is no more toxic than other conventional DMARDs. A meta-analysis of 88 studies on patients who had been treated for at least 12 years showed a discontinuation rate of MTX due to side effects that was lower than for sulfasalazine, gold or D-penicillamine, but slightly higher than for hydroxychloroquine (76). A long-term study of 1681 patients on various standard therapies showed that after four years almost 40% of the initially treated patients were still receiving MTX as monotherapy – more than any other DMARD. The discontinuation rate due to side effects was 16%, bearing in mind that folic acid substitution had not yet been established at that time (47).

In prospective studies on combination therapy, MTX does not show any relevant increased toxicity compared to monotherapy. Although an initial meta-analysis revealed a slightly increased risk of adverse effects with combination therapy, this did not apply to the combinations of MTX with tumor necrosis factor-α inhibitors, sulfasalazine and antimalarials used in practice (23, 27). A more recent meta-analysis of 16 controlled studies (TNF inhibitors, abatacept, tocilizumab and rituximab) also showed no differences in the number of serious adverse events (SAE) and severe infections – compared between patients taking biologics as monotherapy or in combination with MTX (7). A slightly increased rate of side effects was only found in the combination with ciclosporin A (34). The combination of MTX and leflunomide (LEF) also does not seem to be associated with a significant increase in serious adverse events (17), although cases of severe bone marrow and liver toxicity have been described (69) and the LEF product information advises against this combination.

10.2. Predictors of methotrexate toxicity

Factors that could predispose to increased MTX toxicity are female gender and the cumulative MTX dose (3). In the CONCERTO study, women had a higher rate of adverse events (AE) compared to men, with an OR of 1.9 (95% CI 1.1-3.5). In addition, the total number of AEs and infectious AEs increased in a dose-dependent manner (19). The rate of treatment discontinuation increases with age (12), possibly due to reduced renal clearance (4). In long-term analyses, lack of folate supplementation (see below), untreated hyperlipidemia and an increased body mass index predisposed to liver toxicity, while reduced serum albumin was associated with an increased risk of thrombocytopenia (45).

A large number of studies have been devoted to the search for genetic factors for MTX intolerance. Children with trisomy 21 (Down syndrome) have altered folate homeostasis and are more likely to develop toxic MTX effects (33). Due to the interaction of this drug with folic acid and adenosine metabolism, the influences of allelic polymorphisms of these metabolic pathways on MTX tolerance have been investigated (1, 14, 38, 50, 70, 98). The C677T allele of methylene tetrahydrofolate reductase (*MTHFR*) is associated with increased MTX toxicity in the treatment of patients with juvenile idiopathic arthritis (JIA) and psoriatic arthritis (PsA) (20, 88). In contrast, a meta-analysis of 1514 rheumatoid arthritis (RA) patients could not demonstrate an association of C677T with MTX intolerance (54). In European patients, a meta-analysis found that the *MTHFR* polymorphism RFC-1 80G > A (rs1051266) was associated with increased toxicity (68). However, the analysis of gene polymorphisms is of no importance in rheumatological practice.

It was investigated whether therapeutic drug monitoring can reduce the rate of AEs. The level of free MTX is unsuitable for this purpose due to its short half-life (52). However, MTX is stored as polyglutamate in erythrocytes and leukocytes. However, a recent study on large numbers of cases showed a weak association between high MTX polyglutamate levels and elevated liver function parameters. Many other toxicity parameters showed no association or only a trend (100). In addition, changes in MTX polyglutamate levels are too slow to be a meaningful indicator of overdoses or impending AEs (84).

10.3. Gastrointestinal side effects

The most common reported side effects include nausea, vomiting and upper abdominal pain, with a frequency between 10 and 50% (2). The supplementation with folic or folinic acid reduces the occurrence of gastrointestinal side effects (81). The percentage of gastrointestinal intolerance is particularly high if the starting dose is higher than usual (e.g. 25 mg per week) or if the dose is increased rapidly to 25 to 30 mg (93). Nausea occurred less frequently when MTX was started at the same time as low-dose prednisolone therapy (6).

10.3.1. Hepatotoxicity

Temporary elevations in transaminases (TA) can be detected in 13-30% of patients with short-term treatment and in up to half of cases with long-term treatment (71). Increased TA are more common in patients with PsA than with RA (15% vs 8%) (86). These laboratory phenomena cannot always be distinguished from the effect of other medications, in particular from the increase in TA from using diclofenac or other NSAIDs. Concomitant steroid administration may reduce the frequency of increased TA. In an MTX study in which RA patients received blinded steroids or placebo, increased TA were significantly less common when using prednisolone (6). In over 600 patients who received MTX for sarcoidosis, slightly increased TA were only measured in 1.6% – about 60% of them received steroids (9).

In long-term studies, only 4% of patients discontinue MTX due to hepatic side effects (76). The significance of an increase in TA during MTX therapy is questionable: when patients with inflammatory bowel disease whose TA rose when taking MTX continued treatment nevertheless, TA normalized spontaneously in 64%. 10 of the 11 patients from this cohort who underwent a liver biopsy did not have pathological liver histology (31). In addition, liver fibrosis does not correlate with the incidence of increased TA: the closest association was observed between liver fibrosis and cholestasis parameters (11).

The development of liver cirrhosis was long considered a feared side effect of MTX. However, most reports of the development of liver cirrhosis are found in patients who were treated with MTX for psoriasis (66). In the treatment of children with juvenile idiopathic arthritis, hepatotoxicity is of little significance despite the relatively high doses used (49).

According to current knowledge, the hepatic risk is manageable when using MTX for rheumatological indications (8). The incidence of fibrosing liver changes of all degrees of severity lies in the range of 5% after several years of therapy (8). Patients who already had an increase in TA before starting therapy (92), overweight patients and diabetics (11), as well as patients with fatty liver and non-alcoholic steatohepatitis (64) have the highest risk of developing liver damage using MTX. Another predisposing factor is the lack of folic or folinic acid supplementation (8). Data on the frequency of serious structural liver changes vary. The risk of cirrhosis after 5 years was given as 0.1%, but the affected patients also consumed more than 100 g of alcohol per day (!) (94). A meta-analysis determined the frequency of liver fibrosis to be 3% after four years of MTX therapy. In contrast, two other studies that evaluated sequential liver biopsies showed no evidence of irreversible liver damage (76).

10.4. Pulmonary toxicity

Pulmonary toxicity of MTX was first observed during high-dose treatment of leukemia (71). Publications from the 1990s reported case series of MTX-induced pneumonitis in RA patients. One of the larger samples described 27 cases of MTX pneumonitis. The clinical signs consisted mainly of shortness of breath, cough and fever. The mortality rate was 17%. Half of the patients became conspicuous in the first 32 weeks of therapy (51). In 371 patients who were treated with MTX for a median of 4.6 years, cough and shortness of breath led to treatment discontinuation in 4% of cases, although it is doubtful whether these were definitively MTX pneumonitis (47). Case reports of pulmonary toxicity with the combination of MTX and LEF are noteworthy (74). According to older literature data, the incidence of MTX-induced pneumonitis varies between 2% and up to 33% (53). In contrast, a more recent meta-analysis calculates an incidence of only 0.3% (13 cases of 4544 patients treated with MTX) (24). A current prospective study (Cardiovascular Inflammation Reduction Trial, CIRT study) found the same frequency in 2391 MTX patients (83). Pneumonitis has also been described when using other DMARDs, including LEF, AZA and TNF inhibitors (73), so it is questionable whether this is a substance-specific side effect.

The pathogenesis of MTX pneumonitis is only partially understood. Idiosyncratic reactions, non-cardiogenic pulmonary edema, or a hypersensitivity reaction are discussed (53). The promotion of pulmonary infections has also been discussed, but in the meta-analysis mentioned above, the risk of pulmonary infections with MTX treatment was only slightly increased (OR 1.1; CI 1.0-1.2) (24). Pulmonary toxicity is suspected if radiological findings show pulmonary, interstitial or alveolar infiltrates and blood and sputum cultures do not provide any evidence of pathogenic agents. A chest X-ray before starting MTX therapy makes it easier to differentiate between pre-existing and newly occurring pulmonary changes.

There is no convincing evidence in the literature for the induction of interstitial lung disease (ILD) by MTX (10, 25). There is also no evidence that ILD predisposes to increased MTX toxicity (25). On the contrary, MTX therapy in RA reduces the incidence and progression of ILD, so that MTX is not contraindicated in RA patients with this lung disease, but is rather considered helpful (32).

10.5. Hematological toxicity

Treatment with MTX can lead to neutropenia. This can be severe if the elimination of MTX is impaired by renal insufficiency (44). Therefore, even in cases of mildly impaired renal function, the MTX dose must be reduced; if the glomerular filtration rate is below 30 ml/min, MTX is contraindicated (28).

Hematological side effects during MTX treatment are not a common occurrence. Of 165 patients who had been treated with MTX for a median of 75 months, only 4% had abnormal hematological findings. These included three cases of neutropenia and one case each of persistent lymphocytosis and monocytosis (99). In a retrospective analysis, 278 patients had leukopenia of less than 3 Gpt/l in 0.7/100 patient years and thrombocytopenia of less than 100 Gpt/l in 0.3/100 patient years. None of these deviations led to serious complications (102). In the above-mentioned CIRT study, bicytopenia (4%) and pancytopenia (0.5%) were rare during the treatment period of 2.3 years. No pancytopenia was severe, only 3 of 13 of these patients had to permanently discontinue MTX (91).

Risk factors for the development of pancytopenia when using MTX include age over 75 years, renal insufficiency and a pre-existing folic acid deficiency (56). Hypoalbuminemia also predisposes to bone marrow toxicity (12, 56).

An increase in MCV, which is considered a sign of overdose in AZA therapy, is not an indicator of hematological toxicity in MTX treatment (99). Substitution of folic acid after MTX administration prevents the decrease of folate in erythrocytes and reduces the risk of myelotoxicity (41).

10.6. Side effects affecting the skin, mucous membranes and subcutaneous tissue

Dermatological side effects primarily affect the gingiva. These range from poorly healing ulcers to lymphoma-like growths (42), and can be indicators of an overdose (87). A retrospective analysis of 371 patients lists gingivitis as 9% of the side effects leading to discontinuation, but allergic skin reactions as only 2% (47). However, folate substitution was not yet established during the treatment period examined. This can significantly reduce undesirable effects on the mucous membranes (67).

Allergic skin reactions are rare. Their severity ranges from urticaria to leukocytoclastic vasculitis (71), although it is often not easy to clearly assign MTX to the lesions mentioned. Hair loss is observed relatively frequently with MTX, but rarely leads to discontinuation of therapy (47).

In the 1990s, it was claimed that MTX leads to an increased formation of rheumatoid nodules (46, 79). However, this hypothesis has never been prospectively investigated. There is no plausible concept for the pathogenetic substantiation of this assumption. In recent years, this idea has left the spotlight, possibly because rheumatoid nodules are no longer part of the diagnostic criteria and are no longer systematically documented.

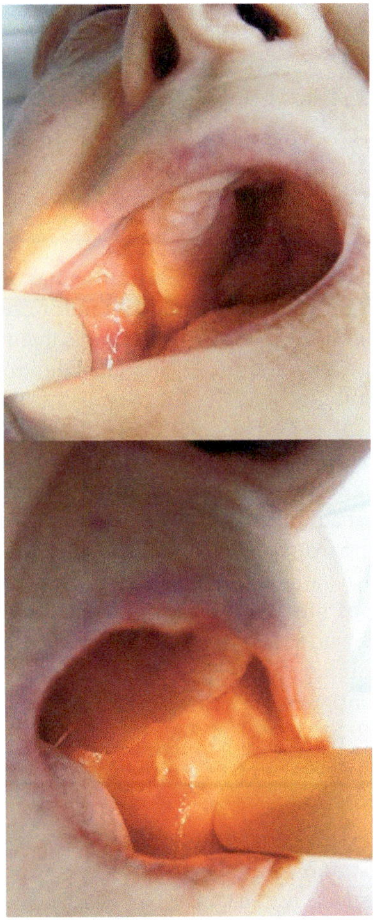

Figure 10.1: Oral ulcers in leukopenia due to MTX accumulation in renal insufficiency.

10.7. Infections

As an immunosuppressive therapy, MTX treatment may be associated with an increased infection rate. However, it is difficult to determine the contribution of MTX to the development of infections, as RA patients are inherently at risk of infection and the influences of previous treatments, steroids and comorbidity must be taken into account. In analyses from the 1990s, the MTX-related relative risk of infection was given as approximately 1.5 (89). More recent database analyses put the risk of infection into perspective (75). Compared to AZA, there were only half as many infectious events in patients with sarcoidosis taking MTX (7 vs 12% in 6 months) (72). However, MTX can weaken the humoral defense, as demonstrated by the evidence of a significantly reduced vaccination response to pneumococcal vaccine when taking MTX (43). Due to a very low rate of joint and prosthesis infections (76), discontinuation of this basic therapeutic agent before surgery is no longer recommended (35). The combination of biologics and MTX does not lead to a significant increase in severe infectious events compared to biologic monotherapy (7). There are different statements on the risk of herpes zoster infections: in addition to a barely relevant increase with MTX (104), an increase of 50% (101) or a doubling of the risk has been described (55).

Patients taking MTX do not develop more severe courses of COVID-19 infection compared to untreated patients or patients treated with TNF inhibitors (103). Based on a small case series and animal experimental data, a certain protective effect of MTX on the course of an infection with the SARS-CoV-2 virus was even found (77). In RA patients, both MTX and glucocorticoids, but especially the combination of both substances, reduced the response to mRNA vaccines (18); an inhibitory influence of MTX on vaccination success was also demonstrable in psoriasis patients (58). However, after a second vaccination with BNT162b2 (Pfizer Biontech), the development of humoral immunity was not impaired by MTX (57).

10.8. Drug interactions

The number of relevant drug interactions of MTX is manageable (90). Of importance is the interaction with trimethoprim-sulfamethoxazole, which, like MTX, acts as a folic acid antagonist. This can induce severe bone marrow complications and the occurrence of pneumonitis (56). In a meta-analysis of 67 pharmacokinetic studies, observational studies and case reports, the interaction between MTX and trimethoprim-sulfamethoxazole was identified as the most important toxic interaction (15). The additive hepatotoxicity using MTX and

INH could also be important (15), especially if the latter is used as tuberculosis prophylaxis in anti-TNF-α therapy.

There are no prospective studies investigating whether the combination of NSAIDs and MTX is associated with increased toxicity. It should be noted that NSAIDs may impair renal function and therefore impair the excretion of MTX (28).

10.9. Carcinogenicity

A meta-analysis confirms that MTX has no relevant carcinogenic potential (76); another retrospective analysis sees the cancer risk for MTX patients as higher than with treatment using other conventional DMARDs or TNF inhibitors (82), especially with regard to non-melanotic skin cancers and solid tumors. The CIRT study found no general increase in tumor incidence in over 2300 patients after three years, but also a higher rate of skin tumors when using MTX, primarily squamous cell carcinomas (HR 3.3; 95% CI 1.6-6.7) (91). When assessing the tumor risk in RA patients, the activity of the underlying disease must be taken into account: RA patients have a higher risk of lymphomas, but a lower risk of colon cancer compared to healthy individuals, which is attributed to the influence of NSAIDs (85). Disease activity itself, rather than its treatment, appears to be the main factor contributing to the increased risk of lymphoma (5).

10.10. Teratogenicity and pregnancy

MTX is used for the drug induction of abortions and is embryotoxic in doses used in chemotherapy (95). The MTX-typical embryopathy (fetal aminopterin syndrome) after high-dose exposure is characterized by musculoskeletal and craniofacial malformations (21). The rate of miscarriage is also significantly increased in women with rheumatic diseases who become pregnant while taking MTX. Malformations occur more frequently, but not the typical picture of the above-mentioned embryopathy (95). In contrast, in over 300 patients who stopped taking MTX before conception, the miscarriage and malformation rates were comparable to those of a control group (95). The duration of MTX treatment had no influence on the conception rate, although patients who became pregnant more than a year after stopping MTX had taken the drug for longer than patients who conceived more quickly (1.7 vs. 3.2 years) (65). However, the age of the patients may have had an influence as a confounding factor here. A recent meta-analysis found no delaying effect of MTX on the time to conception (26). There is consensus that MTX should also be avoided during breastfeeding (13).

Children of fathers who took MTX in doses up to a maximum of 30 mg per week do not have an increased risk of malformations (96), premature birth or low birth weight (59).

10.11. Rate of side effects depending on the route of administration and concomitant medication

MTX is nowadays mainly administered subcutaneously. The route of administration has no influence on its tolerability (16, 37). A randomized double-blind study comparing oral and subcutaneous administration found only marginal differences in the tolerability of MTX. The overall rate of side effects and the rate of serious side effects were slightly higher with subcutaneous administration, but diarrhea and abdominal pain were more common with oral administration (16). In a real-life study, switching from oral to subcutaneous administration in RA patients improved substance adherence, quality of life and disease control (80). 86% of patients who were switched from oral to subcutaneous administration due to side effects or ineffectivity continued MTX therapy after one year (78).

Dividing the oral MTX dose into two single doses has no relevant impact on the tolerability of the drug (36).

The supplementation of folic acid after MTX administration was controversial for a long time because it was feared that MTX would lose its effectivity (48, 61). However, a cohort study showed that over 70% of patients continued to take MTX after 5 years of folic acid supplementation; without this co-medication, the same rate was 30% (39). This success was mainly attributed to lower hepatotoxicity. Folate supplementation reduced the frequency of TA increases to more than three times the norm by almost 90% (40). In addition, the administration of folic acid significantly improved the gastrointestinal tolerance of MTX (62, 63). In addition, folic acid reduces the homocysteine levels increased by MTX. Homocysteine is associated with the development of arteriosclerotic vascular changes (60).

The combination of MTX with low-dose steroids may also lead to improved tolerability of MTX. In the CAMERA study, which combined MTX with 10 mg prednisolone or placebo, significantly fewer patients had nausea with prednisolone than with placebo (23% vs 43%); the same applied to the frequency of stomatitis (9% vs 18%) and TA elevation (15% vs 33%) (6).

10.12. Summary

According to current guidelines, MTX is the recognized drug for the initial treatment of RA (29). The very good long-term safety and tolerability is supported by data showing that MTX therapy for RA patients has advantages for long-term survival (22) and the frequency of cardiovascular events (97). It is therefore likely that MTX will retain its important role in treatment of rheumatic diseases in the coming years.

10.13. References

1. Aggarwal P, Naik S, Mishra KP et al. (2006) Correlation between methotrexate efficacy & toxicity with C677T polymorphism of the methylenetetrahydrofolate gene in rheumatoid arthritis patients on folate supplementation. The Indian Journal of Medical Research 124: 521-526

2. Albrecht K, Muller-Ladner U (2010) Side effects and management of side effects of methotrexate in rheumatoid arthritis. Clinical and Experimental Rheumatology 28:S95-101

3. Amital H, Arnson Y, Chodick G et al. (2009) Hepatotoxicity rates do not differ in patients with rheumatoid arthritis and psoriasis treated with methotrexate. Rheumatology (Oxford) 48:1107-1110

4. Arakawa Y, Arakawa A, Vural S et al. (2019) Renal clearance and intracellular half-life essentially determine methotrexate toxicity: A case series. JAAD Case Reports 5:98-100

5. Baecklund E, Iliadou A, Askling J et al. (2006) Association of chronic inflammation, not its treatment, with increased lymphoma risk in rheumatoid arthritis. Arthritis and Rheumatism 54:692-701

6. Bakker MF, Jacobs JW, Welsing PM et al. (2012) Low-dose prednisone inclusion in a methotrexate-based, tight control strategy for early rheumatoid arthritis: a randomized trial. Annals of Internal Medicine 156:329-339

7. Baradat C, Degboé Y, Constantin A et al. (2017) No impact of concomitant methotrexate use on serious adverse event and serious infection risk in patients with rheumatoid arthritis treated with bDMARDs: a systematic literature review and meta-analysis. RMD Open 3: e000352

8. Bath RK, Brar NK, Forouhar FA et al. (2014) A review of methotrexate-associated hepatotoxicity. Journal of Digestive Diseases 15:517-524

9. Baughman RP, Cremers JP, Harmon M et al. (2020) Methotrexate in sarcoidosis: hematologic and hepatic toxicity encountered in a large cohort over a six year period. Sarcoidosis Vasc Diffuse Lung Dis 37:e2020001

10. Belzunegui J, Intxausti JJ, De Dios JR et al. (2001) Absence of pulmonary fibrosis in patients with psoriatic arthritis treated with weekly low-dose methotrexate. Clinical and Experimental Rheumatology 19:727-730

11. Berends MA, Snoek J, De Jong EM et al. (2006) Liver injury in long-term methotrexate treatment in psoriasis is relatively infrequent. Alimentary Pharmacology & Therapeutics 24: 805-811

12. Bernatsky S, Ehrmann Feldman D (2008) Discontinuation of methotrexate therapy in older patients with newly diagnosed rheumatoid arthritis: analysis of administrative health databases in Quebec, Canada. Drugs & Aging 25:879-884

13. Birru Talabi M, Clowse MEB (2020) Antirheumatic medications in pregnancy and breastfeeding. Current Opinion in Rheumatology 32:238-246

14. Bohanec Grabar P, Logar D, Lestan B et al. (2008) Genetic determinants of methotrexate toxicity in rheumatoid arthritis patients: a study of polymorphisms affecting methotrexate transport and folate metabolism. European Journal of Clinical Pharmacology 64:1057-1068

15. Bourre-Tessier J, Haraoui B (2010) Methotrexate drug interactions in the treatment of rheumatoid arthritis: a systematic review. The Journal of Rheumatology 37:1416-1421

16. Braun J, Kastner P, Flaxenberg P et al. (2008) Comparison of the clinical efficacy and safety of subcutaneous versus oral administration of methotrexate in patients with active rheumatoid arthritis: results of a six-month, multicenter, randomized, double-blind, controlled, phase IV trial. Arthritis and Rheumatism 58:73-81

17. Bredemeier M, Ranza R, Kakehasi AM et al. (2021) Safety of the methotrexate-leflunomide combination in rheumatoid arthritis: results of a multicentric, registry-based, cohort study (BiobadaBrasil). The Journal of Rheumatology 48:1519-1527

18. Bugatti S, De Stefano L, Balduzzi S et al. (2021) Methotrexate and glucocorticoids, but not anticytokine therapy, impair the immunogenicity of a single dose of the BNT162b2 mRNA COVID-19 vaccine in patients with chronic inflammatory arthritis. Annals of the Rheumatic Diseases 80:1635-1638

19. Burmester GR, Kaeley GS, Kavanaugh AF et al. (2017) Treatment efficacy and methotrexate-related toxicity in patients with rheumatoid arthritis receiving methotrexate in combination with adalimumab. RMD Open 3:e000465

20. Chandran V, Siannis F, Rahman P et al. (2010) Folate pathway enzyme gene polymorphisms and the efficacy and toxicity of methotrexate in psoriatic arthritis. The Journal of Rheumatology 37:1508-1512

21. Chapa JB, Hibbard JU, Weber EM et al. (2003) Prenatal diagnosis of methotrexate embryopathy. Obstetrics and Gynecology 101:1104-1107

22. Choi HK, Hernan MA, Seeger JD et al. (2002) Methotrexate and mortality in patients with rheumatoid arthritis: a prospective study. Lancet 359:1173-1177

23. Choy EH, Smith C, Dore CJ et al. (2005) A meta-analysis of the efficacy and toxicity of combining disease-modifying antirheumatic drugs in rheumatoid arthritis based on patient withdrawal. Rheumatology (Oxford) 44:1414-1421

24. Conway R, Low C, Coughlan RJ et al. (2014) Methotrexate and lung disease in rheumatoid arthritis: a meta-analysis of randomized controlled trials. Arthritis Rheumatol 66:803-812

25. Dawson JK, Graham DR, Desmond J et al. (2002) Investigation of the chronic pulmonary effects of low-dose oral methotrexate in patients with rheumatoid arthritis: a prospective study incorporating HRCT scanning and pulmonary function tests. Rheumatology (Oxford) 41: 262-267

26. De Cock D, Brants L, Soenen I et al. (2020) A systematic review on the effect of DMARDs on fertility in rheumatoid arthritis. Seminars in Arthritis and Rheumatism 50:873-878

27. Elkayam O, Yaron M, Zhukovsky G et al. (1997) Toxicity profile of dual methotrexate combinations with gold, hydroxychloroquine, sulphasalazine and minocycline in rheumatoid arthritis patients. Rheumatology international 17:49-53

28. Erdbrugger U, De Groot K (2011) [Is methotrexate nephrotoxic? Dose-dependency, comorbidities and comedication]. Zeitschrift fur Rheumatologie 70:549-552

29. Fiehn C, Holle J, Iking-Konert C et al. (2018) [S2e guideline: treatment of rheumatoid arthritis with disease-modifying drugs]. Zeitschrift fur Rheumatologie 77:35-53

30. Fleisher M (1993) Antifolate analogs: mechanism of action, analytical methodology, and clinical efficacy. Therapeutic Drug Monitoring 15:521-526

31. Fournier MR, Klein J, Minuk GY et al. (2010) Changes in liver biochemistry during methotrexate use for inflammatory bowel disease. The American Journal of Gastroenterology 105:1620-1626

32. Fragoulis GE, Nikiphorou E, Larsen J et al. (2019) Methotrexate-associated pneumonitis and rheumatoid arthritis-interstitial lung disease: Current concepts for the diagnosis and treatment. Frontiers in Medicine 6

33. Funk RS, Talib NJ, Zimmerman KO et al. (2020) Altered folate homeostasis in children with down syndrome: A potential basis for enhanced methotrexate toxicity. The Journal of Pediatrics 221:235-239

34. Gerards AH, Landewe RB, Prins AP et al. (2003) Cyclosporin A monotherapy versus cyclosporin A and methotrexate combination therapy in patients with early rheumatoid arthritis: a double blind randomised placebo controlled trial. Annals of the Rheumatic Diseases 62:291-296

35. Goodman SM (2015) Optimizing perioperative outcomes for older patients with rheumatoid arthritis undergoing arthroplasty: emphasis on medication management. Drugs & Aging 32:361-369

36. Goodman SM, Cronstein BN, Bykerk VP (2015) Outcomes related to methotrexate dose and route of administration in patients with rheumatoid arthritis: a systematic literature review. Clinical and Experimental Rheumatology 33: 272-278

37. Hazlewood GS, Thorne JC, Pope JE et al. (2015) The comparative effectiveness of oral versus subcutaneous methotrexate for the treatment of early rheumatoid arthritis. Annals of the Rheumatic Diseases

38. Hider SL, Thomson W, Mack LF et al. (2008) Polymorphisms within the adenosine receptor 2a gene are associated with adverse events in RA patients treated with MTX. Rheumatology (Oxford) 47:1156-1159

39. Hoekstra M, Van De Laar MA, Bernelot Moens HJ et al. (2003) Longterm observational study of methotrexate use in a Dutch cohort of 1022 patients with rheumatoid arthritis. The Journal of Rheumatology 30:2325-2329

40. Hoekstra M, Van Ede AE, Haagsma CJ et al. (2003) Factors associated with toxicity, final dose, and efficacy of methotrexate in patients with rheumatoid arthritis. Annals of the Rheumatic Diseases 62:423-426

41. Hornung N, Ellingsen T, Stengaard-Pedersen K et al. (2004) Folate, homocysteine, and cobalamin status in patients with rheumatoid arthritis treated with methotrexate, and the effect of low dose folic acid supplement. The Journal of Rheumatology 31:2374-2381

42. Kalantzis A, Marshman Z, Falconer DT et al. (2005) Oral effects of low-dose methotrexate treatment. Oral Surgery, Oral Medicine, Oral Pathology, Oral Radiology, and Endodontics 100:52-62

43. Kapetanovic MC, Saxne T, Sjoholm A et al. (2006) Influence of methotrexate, TNF blockers and prednisolone on antibody responses to pneumococcal polysaccharide vaccine in patients with rheumatoid arthritis. Rheumatology (Oxford) 45:106-111

44. Karie S, Gandjbakhch F, Janus N et al. (2008) Kidney disease in RA patients: prevalence and implication on RA-related drugs management: the MATRIX study. Rheumatology (Oxford) 47:350-354

45. Kent PD, Luthra HS, Michet C, Jr. (2004) Risk factors for methotrexate-induced abnormal laboratory monitoring results in patients with rheumatoid arthritis. The Journal of Rheumatology 31:1727-1731

46. Kerstens PJ, Boerbooms AM, Jeurissen ME et al. (1992) Accelerated nodulosis during low dose methotrexate therapy for rheumatoid arthritis. An analysis of ten cases. The Journal of Rheumatology 19:867-871

47. Keysser M, Keysser G, Keysser C (1999) Long-term application of disease modifying antirheumatic drugs (DMARD). A single-center, observational study of 1681 patients with rheumatoid arthritis (RA). Zeitschrift fur Rheumatologie 58: 267-276

48. Khanna D, Park GS, Paulus HE et al. (2005) Reduction of the efficacy of methotrexate by the use of folic acid: post hoc analysis from two randomized controlled studies. Arthritis and Rheumatism 52:3030-3038

49. Kocharla L, Taylor J, Weiler T et al. (2009) Monitoring methotrexate toxicity in juvenile idiopathic arthritis. The Journal of Rheumatology 36:2813-2818

50. Kooloos WM, Wessels JA, Van Der Straaten T et al. (2010) Functional polymorphisms and methotrexate treatment outcome in recent-onset rheumatoid arthritis. Pharmacogenomics 11:163-175

51. Kremer JM, Alarcon GS, Weinblatt ME et al. (1997) Clinical, laboratory, radiographic, and histopathologic features of methotrexate-associated lung injury in patients with rheumatoid arthritis: a multicenter study with literature review. Arthritis and Rheumatism 40: 1829-1837

52. Lafforgue P, Monjanel-Mouterde S, Durand A et al. (1995) Lack of correlation between pharmacokinetics and efficacy of low dose methotrexate in patients with rheumatoid arthritis. The Journal of Rheumatology 22: 844-849

53. Lateef O, Shakoor N, Balk RA (2005) Methotrexate pulmonary toxicity. Expert Opinion on Drug Safety 4: 723-730

54. Lee YH, Song GG (2010) Associations between the C677T and A1298C polymorphisms of MTHFR and the efficacy and toxicity of methotrexate in rheumatoid arthritis: a meta-analysis. Clinical Drug Investigation 30:101-108

55. Liao TL, Chen YM, Liu HJ et al. (2017) Risk and severity of herpes zoster in patients with rheumatoid arthritis receiving different immunosuppressive medications: a case-control study in Asia. BMJ Open 7: e014032

56. Lim AY, Gaffney K, Scott DG (2005) Methotrexate-induced pancytopenia: serious and under-reported? Our experience of 25 cases in 5 years. Rheumatology (Oxford) 44:1051-1055

57. Mahil SK, Bechman K, Raharja A et al. (2022) Humoral and cellular immunogenicity to a second dose of COVID-19 vaccine BNT162b2 in people receiving methotrexate or targeted immunosuppression: a longitudinal cohort study. Lancet Rheumatol 4:e42-e52

58. Mahil SK, Bechman K, Raharja A et al. (2021) The effect of methotrexate and targeted immunosuppression on humoral and cellular immune responses to the COVID-19 vaccine BNT162b2: a cohort study. Lancet Rheumatol 3:e627-e637

59. Meserve J, Luo J, Zhu W et al. (2021) Paternal exposure to immunosuppressive and/or biologic agents and birth outcomes in patients with immune-mediated inflammatory diseases. Gastroenterology 161:107-115. e103

60. Morgan SL, Baggott JE (2010) Folate supplementation during methotrexate therapy for rheumatoid arthritis. Clinical and Experimental Rheumatology 28:S102-109

61. Morgan SL, Baggott JE, Alarcon GS (1997) Methotrexate in rheumatoid arthritis: folate supplementation should always be given. BioDrugs: Clinical Immunotherapeutics, Biopharmaceuticals and Gene Therapy 8:164-175

62. Morgan SL, Baggott JE, Vaughn WH et al. (1994) Supplementation with folic acid during methotrexate therapy for rheumatoid arthritis. A double-blind, placebo-controlled trial. Annals of Internal Medicine 121:833-841

63. Morgan SL, Baggott JE, Vaughn WH et al. (1990) The effect of folic acid supplementation on the toxicity of low-dose methotrexate in patients with rheumatoid arthritis. Arthritis and Rheumatism 33:9-18

64. Mori S, Arima N, Ito M et al. (2020) Incidence, predictive factors and severity of methotrexate-related liver injury in rheumatoid arthritis: a longitudinal cohort study. Rheumatol Adv Pract 4:rkaa020

65. Nagafuchi H, Goto Y, Kiyokawa T et al. (2021) Pregnancy outcomes in patients with rheumatoid arthritis who discontinue methotrexate treatment to conceive. Clinical Rheumatology

66. Nyfors A, Hopwood D (1977) Liver ultrastructure in psoriatics related to methotrexate therapy. 1. A prospective study of findings in hepatocytes from 24 patients before and after methotrexate treatment. Acta pathologica et microbiologica Scandinavica. Section A, Pathology 85:787-800

67. Ortiz Z, Shea B, Suarez Almazor M et al. (2000) Folic acid and folinic acid for reducing side effects in patients receiving methotrexate for rheumatoid arthritis. The Cochrane Database of Systematic Reviews:CD000951

68. Qiu Q, Huang J, Lin Y et al. (2017) Polymorphisms and pharmacogenomics for the toxicity of methotrexate monotherapy in patients with rheumatoid arthritis: A systematic review and meta-analysis. Medicine 96:e6337

69. Qu C, Lu Y, Liu W (2017) Severe bone marrow suppression accompanying pulmonary infection and hemorrhage of the digestive tract associated with leflunomide and low-dose methotrexate combination therapy. J Pharmacol Pharmacother 8:35-37

70. Ranganathan P (2006) Association of methotrexate effects and single-nucleotide polymorphisms in the folate pathway in rheumatoid arthritis: comment on the article by Wessels et al. Arthritis and Rheumatism 54:3372; author reply 3372-3373

71. Rau R, Herborn G (2004) Benefit and risk of methotrexate treatment in rheumatoid arthritis. Clinical and Experimental Rheumatology 22:S83-94

72. Rossides M, Kullberg S, Di Giuseppe D et al. (2021) Infection risk in sarcoidosis patients treated with methotrexate compared to azathioprine: A retrospective 'target trial' emulated with Swedish real-world data. Respirology 26:452-460

73. Roubille C, Haraoui B (2014) Interstitial lung diseases induced or exacerbated by DMARDS and biologic agents in rheumatoid arthritis: a systematic literature review. Seminars in Arthritis and Rheumatism 43:613-626

74. Rutanen J, Kononoff A, Arstila L et al. (2014) Five cases of interstitial lung disease after leflunomide was combined with methotrexate therapy. Scandinavian Journal of Rheumatology 43:254-256

75. Sakai R, Komano Y, Tanaka M et al. (2011) The REAL database reveals no significant risk of serious infection during treatment with a methotrexate dose of more than 8 mg/week in patients with rheumatoid arthritis. Modern rheumatology / the Japan Rheumatism Association 21:444-448

76. Salliot C, Van Der Heijde D (2009) Long-term safety of methotrexate monotherapy in patients with rheumatoid arthritis: a systematic literature research. Annals of the Rheumatic Diseases 68:1100-1104

77. Schälter F, Dürholz K, Bucci L et al. (2021) Does methotrexate influence COVID-19 infection? Case series and mechanistic data. Arthritis Research & Therapy 23: 166

78. Scott DG, Claydon P, Ellis C (2014) Retrospective evaluation of continuation rates following a switch to subcutaneous methotrexate in rheumatoid arthritis patients failing to respond to or tolerate oral methotrexate: the MENTOR study. Scandinavian Journal of Rheumatology 43:470-476

79. Segal R, Caspi D, Tishler M et al. (1988) Accelerated nodulosis and vasculitis during methotrexate therapy for rheumatoid arthritis. Arthritis and Rheumatism 31: 1182-1185

80. Senbel E, Tropé S, Herman-Demars H et al. (2021) Benefits of switch from oral to subcutaneous route on adherence to

methotrexate in patients with rheumatoid arthritis in real life setting. Patient Preference and Adherence 15:751-760

81. Shea B, Swinden MV, Ghogomu ET et al. (2014) Folic acid and folinic acid for reducing side effects in patients receiving methotrexate for rheumatoid arthritis. The Journal of Rheumatology 41:1049-1060

82. Solomon DH, Kremer JM, Fisher M et al. (2014) Comparative cancer risk associated with methotrexate, other non-biologic and biologic disease-modifying anti-rheumatic drugs. Seminars in Arthritis and Rheumatism 43:489-497

83. Sparks JA, Dellaripa PF, Glynn RJ et al. (2020) Pulmonary adverse events in patients receiving low-dose methotrexate in the randomized, double-blind, placebo-controlled cardiovascular inflammation reduction trial. Arthritis Rheumatol 72: 2065-2071

84. Stamp LK, Barclay M (2014) Therapeutic drug monitoring in rheumatic diseases: utile or futile? Rheumatology (Oxford) 53:988-997

85. Symmons DP, Silman AJ (2004) Anti-tumor necrosis factor alpha therapy and the risk of lymphoma in rheumatoid arthritis: no clear answer. Arthritis and Rheumatism 50:1703-1706

86. Tilling L, Townsend S, David J (2006) Methotrexate and hepatic toxicity in rheumatoid arthritis and psoriatic arthritis. Clinical Drug Investigation 26:55-62

87. Troeltzsch M, Von Blohn G, Kriegelstein S et al. (2013) Oral mucositis in patients receiving low-dose methotrexate therapy for rheumatoid arthritis: report of 2 cases and literature review. Oral Surgery, Oral Medicine, Oral Pathology and Oral Radiology 115:e28-33

88. Tukova J, Chladek J, Hroch M et al. (2010) 677TT genotype is associated with elevated risk of methotrexate (MTX) toxicity in juvenile idiopathic arthritis: treatment outcome, erythrocyte concentrations of MTX and folates, and MTHFR polymorphisms. The Journal of Rheumatology 37:2180-2186

89. Van Der Veen MJ, Van Der Heide A, Kruize AA et al. (1994) Infection rate and use of antibiotics in patients with rheumatoid arthritis treated with methotrexate. Annals of the Rheumatic Diseases 53:224-228

90. Van Roon EN, Van Den Bemt PM, Jansen TL et al. (2009) An evidence-based assessment of the clinical significance of drug-drug interactions between disease-modifying antirheumatic drugs and non-antirheumatic drugs according to rheumatologists and pharmacists. Clinical Therapeutics 31:1737-1746

91. Vanni KMM, Berliner N, Paynter NP et al. (2020) Adverse effects of low-dose methotrexate in a randomized double-blind placebo-controlled trial: Adjudicated hematologic and skin cancer outcomes in the cardiovascular inflammation reduction trial. ACR Open Rheumatol 2:697-704

92. Verstappen SM, Bakker MF, Heurkens AH et al. (2010) Adverse events and factors associated with toxicity in patients with early rheumatoid arthritis treated with methotrexate tight control therapy: the CAMERA study. Annals of the rheumatic diseases 69:1044-1048

93. Visser K, Van Der Heijde D (2009) Optimal dosage and route of administration of methotrexate in rheumatoid arthritis: a systematic review of the literature. Annals of the Rheumatic Diseases 68:1094-1099

94. Walker AM, Funch D, Dreyer NA et al. (1993) Determinants of serious liver disease among patients receiving low-dose methotrexate for rheumatoid arthritis. Arthritis and Rheumatism 36:329-335

95. Weber-Schoendorfer C, Chambers C, Wacker E et al. (2014) Pregnancy outcome after methotrexate treatment for rheumatic disease prior to or during early pregnancy: a prospective multicenter cohort study. Arthritis Rheumatol 66: 1101-1110

96. Weber-Schoendorfer C, Hoeltzenbein M, Wacker E et al. (2014) No evidence for an increased risk of adverse pregnancy outcome after paternal low-dose methotrexate: an observational cohort study. Rheumatology (Oxford) 53:757-763

97. Wei L, Macdonald TM, Walker BR (2004) Taking glucocorticoids by prescription is associated with subsequent cardiovascular disease. Annals of Internal Medicine 141:764-770

98. Wessels JA, Kooloos WM, De Jonge R et al. (2006) Relationship between genetic variants in the adenosine pathway and outcome of methotrexate treatment in patients with recent-onset rheumatoid arthritis. Arthritis and Rheumatism 54:2830-2839

99. White DH, Chapman PT, O'donnell JL et al. (2010) Lack of association between elevated mean red cell volume and haematological toxicity in patients receiving long-term methotrexate for rheumatoid arthritis. Internal Medicine Journal 40:561-565

100. Xu C, Selhub J, Jacques P et al. (2021) Adverse effects related to methotrexate polyglutamate levels: adjudicated results from the cardiovascular inflammation reduction trial. Rheumatology (Oxford) 60:2963-2968

101. Yamaguchi R, Tanaka E, Nakajima A et al. (2021) Risk of herpes zoster in patients with rheumatoid arthritis in the biologics era from 2011 to 2015 and its association with methotrexate, biologics, and corticosteroids. Modern Rheumatology

102. Yazici Y (2010) Long-term safety of methotrexate in the treatment of rheumatoid arthritis. Clinical and Experimental Rheumatology 28:S65-67

103. Yousaf A, Gayam S, Feldman S et al. (2021) Clinical outcomes of COVID-19 in patients taking tumor necrosis factor inhibitors or methotrexate: A multicenter research network study. Journal of the American Academy of Dermatology 84:70-75

104. Zhang N, Wilkinson S, Riaz M et al. (2012) Does methotrexate increase the risk of varicella or herpes zoster infection in patients with rheumatoid arthritis? A systematic literature review. Clinical and Experimental Rheumatology 30:962-971

11. Methotrexate and family planning

The professional discussions surrounding the topic of methotrexate (MTX), conception, pregnancy and breastfeeding have increased significantly in recent years.

Fertility is not affected by low-dose MTX use in women, and in men, oligospermia has only been described in very few isolated cases and was usually reversible (1).

Typical malformations with MTX treatment in the first trimester are neural tube defects as well as anomalies of the skull and skeleton. A critical phase for malformations is postulated between the 6th and 8th week of gestation. MTX embryopathies after low-dose treatment (10-30 mg per week) are limited to a few isolated cases. In a large prospective multicenter observational study, the pregnancy courses of women who took MTX (≤30 mg per week) either after conception or within 12 weeks before conception were examined and compared with pregnancies in women with similar diseases and a group of women without autoimmune diseases (neither of the two groups had received MTX) (2). The study included 324 MTX-exposed pregnancies (188 exposed after and 136 exposed, each before conception), 459 disease-matched controls and 1,107 controls without autoimmune diseases. In the cohort with MTX therapy after conception, the incidence of spontaneous miscarriage was 43% (95% CI 29-59) and was thus significantly higher than in both comparison groups. The risk of major congenital malformations (7 of 106 [7%]) was increased both compared to the cohort of women without autoimmune diseases (29 of 1,001 [3%]) (OR 3.1; 95% CI 1.0-9.5) and the disease-adjusted cohort (14 of 393 [4%]) (OR 1.8; 95% CI 0.6-5.7). None of the malformations could be clearly attributed to MTX embryopathy. Neither the incidence of spontaneous miscarriages (14%; 95% CI 8.0-25) nor the risk of major birth defects (4 of 114 [4%]) was increased in the preconception cohort. The rates of elective abortions were increased in both MTX-exposed cohorts. There were no other significant differences between the groups in other endpoints of the study. The authors' important conclusion was that low-dose MTX use after conception is associated with an increased risk of major birth defects and spontaneous miscarriages, but that such evidence was not found for preconception exposure.

Experience with low-dose therapy in the second or third trimester has not yet been documented. Like other cytotoxic drugs, MTX can lead to intrauterine growth retardation, myelosuppression and, very rarely, intrauterine fetal death when used as part a treatment regime for malignant tumors.

11.1. Planning a pregnancy

When planning a pregnancy, MTX must be switched to a safer antirheumatic. It is recommended to stop MTX one to three months before conception (3, 4). Three months is also adequate in order to observe the effectivity and tolerability after a change. When MTX is stopped, higher-dose folic acid substitution should be commenced and continued during pregnancy. There are no validated recommendations regarding the dosing of folic acid. 5 mg folic acid per day [oral] was recently recommended. If necessary, folic acid levels should be tested.

11.2. Conception

A systematic literature search included 17 studies (n=1508 exposed pregnancies) and could not show an association between paternal low-dose MTX use and negative pregnancy outcomes (1). A prospective study of a total of 114 pregnancies with paternal MTX exposure (at or up to three months before conception, dose 7.5-30 mg per week) described no increased risk of malformations, spontaneous miscarriages, premature births or lower birth weight compared to 412 non-exposed pregnancies (5).

> Recommendation: A decision to discontinue treatment must be weighed against the possible effects on paternal disease activity. Current recommendations do not advise discontinuing MTX during preconception if there is an appropriate medical indication for its use (6, 7).

11.3. Consequences of (accidental) use during pregnancy

MTX should be stopped immediately or switched to a safer antirheumatic drug. Folic acid should be administered (5 mg folic acid per day) and a detailed ultrasound investigation should be offered. If low-dose treatment is (accidentally) continued into the first trimester, the risk of malformations appears to be 6-8%. The risk of an early miscarriage is significantly increased.

11.4. Breastfeeding

Breastfeeding is not recommended while taking MTX as there is little data available. A case report describes a 34-year-old RA patient who developed a severe flare-up while breastfeeding despite treatment with cortisone, HCQ and SSZ. The patient breastfed her baby, who was 5 months old at the time, for a further 9 months while on treatment with MTX (25 mg per week subcutaneously). The breast milk contained minimal concentrations, and no clinical symptoms were observed in the child (8).

11.5. References

1. Bermas B. Paternal safety of anti-rheumatic medications. Best Pract Res Clin Obstet Gynaecol 2020;64:77-84.

2. Weber-Schoendorfer C, Chambers C, Wacker E, Beghin D, Bernard N; Network of French Pharmacovigilance Centers, Shechtman S, Johnson D, Cuppers-Maarschalkerweerd B, Pistelli A, Clementi M, Winterfeld U, Eleftheriou G, Pupco A, Kao K, Malm H, Elefant E, Koren G, Vial T, Ornoy A, Meister R, Schaefer C. Pregnancy outcome after methotrexate treatment for rheumatic disease prior to or during early pregnancy: a prospective multicenter cohort study. Arthritis Rheumatol 2014; 66(5):1101-1010.

3. Götestam Skorpen C, Hoeltzenbein M, Tincani A, Fischer-Betz R, Elefant E, Chambers C, da Silva J, Nelson-Piercy C, Cetin I, Costedoat-Chalumeau N, Dolhain R, Förger F, Khamashta M, Ruiz-Irastorza G, Zink A, Vencovsky J, Cutolo M, Caeyers N, Zumbühl C, Østensen M. The EULAR points to consider for use of antirheumatic drugs before pregnancy, and during pregnancy and lactation. Ann Rheum Dis 2016; 75(5):795-810.

4. Flint J, Panchal S, Hurrell A, van de Venne M, Gayed M, Schreiber K, Arthanari S, Cunningham J, Flanders L, Moore L, Crossley A, Purushotham N, Desai A, Piper M, Nisar M, Khamashta M, Williams D, Gordon C, Giles I; BSR and BHPR Standards, Guidelines and Audit Working Group. BSR and BHPR guideline on prescribing drugs in pregnancy and breastfeeding-Part I: standard and biologic disease modifying anti-rheumatic drugs and corticosteroids. Rheumatology (Oxford) 2016; 55(9):1693-1697.

5. Weber-Schoendorfer C, Hoeltzenbein M, Wacker E, Meister R, Schaefer C. No evidence for an increased risk of adverse pregnancy outcome after paternal low-dose methotrexate: an observational cohort study. Rheumatology (Oxford) 2014; 53(4):757-763.

6. Sammaritano LR, Bermas BL, Chakravarty EE, Chambers C, Clowse MEB, Lockshin MD, Marder W, Guyatt G, Branch DW, Buyon J, Christopher-Stine L, Crow-Hercher R, Cush J, Druzin M, Kavanaugh A, Laskin CA, Plante L, Salmon J, Simard J, Somers EC, Steen V, Tedeschi SK, Vinet E, White CW, Yazdany J, Barbhaiya M, Bettendorf B, Eudy A, Jayatilleke A, Shah AA, Sullivan N, Tarter LL, BirruTalabi M, Turgunbaev M, Turner A, D'Anci KE. American College of Rheumatology Guideline for the Management of Reproductive Health in Rheumatic and Musculoskeletal Diseases. Arthritis Rheumatol 2020;72(4):529-556.

7. Fischer-Betz R, Späthling-Mestekemper S. Pregnancy and rheumatic diseases. Z Rheumatol 2020;79(1):55-73.

8. Thorne JC, Nadarajah T, Moretti M, Ito S. Methotrexate use in a breastfeeding patient with rheumatoid arthritis. J Rheumatol 2014;41(11):2332.

12. Abbreviations

ABC	Abatacept
ACR	American College of Rheumatology
ADA	Adalimumab
ADL	Acivities of daily life
ADM	Adalimumab
AF	Auranofin
AICAR	Aminoimidazole carboxyamido-ribonucleotide
ALAT	Alanin aminotransferase (= GPT: Glutamate pyruvate transaminase)
AP	Alkaline phosphatase
ASAT	Aspartate aminotransferase (= GOT: Glutamate oxalacetate transaminase)
ATM	Aurothiomalate
Au	Gold
AUC	Area under the curve
AWMF	Association of scientific medical societies in Germany
AZA	Azathioprine
BAR	Baricitinib
bDMARD	Biological disease-modifying anti-rheumatic drug
BSA	Body surface area
CARRA	Childhood Arthritis and Rheumatology Research Alliance
CCP	Cyclic citrulline peptide
CEZ	Certolizumab
CI	Confidence interval
CIP	Cyclophosphamide
CNS	Central nervous system
CQ	Chloroquin
CRP	C-reactive protein
CS	Circumscript scleroderma
CsA	Ciclosporin A
csDMARD	Conventional synthetic disease-modifying anti-rheumatic drug
CZP	Certolizumab pegol
DAS	Disease activity score
dcSSc	Diffuse cutaneous systemic sclerosis
DGVS	German society for gastroenterology, digestive and metabolic diseases
DHF	Dihydrofolate
DHFR	Dihydrofolate reductase
DM	Dermatomyositis
DMARD	Disease-modifying anti-rheumatic drug
EAA	Enthesitis-associated arthritis
ECCO	European Crohn's and Colitis Organisation
EGPA	Eosinophilic granulomatosis with polyangiitis (formerly Churg-Strauss syndrome)
ES	Erosion score
ESR	Erythrocyte sedimentation rate
ETA	Etanercept
EULAR	European League Against Rheumatism
extOA	Extended oligoarthritis
FAICAR	Formyl-AICAR
FDA	Food and drug administration
FFbH	Hannover functional questionnaire
FIL	Filgotinib
FPGS	Folyl polyglutamate synthetase
FR-β	Folate receptor beta
GC	Glucocorticoids
GFR	Glomerular filtration rate
GOM	Golimumab
GPA	Granulomatosis with polyangiitis (formerly Wegener's disease)
Gpt	Giga particles (=10^9 particles)
γ-GT	gamma-glutamyl transferase
GLM	Golimumab
GTP	Guanosine triphosphate
HADA	Human anti-drug antibodies
HAQ-DI	Health assessment questionnaire disability index
Hb	Hemoglobin
HCQ	Hydroxychloroquine
Hk	Hematocrit
HR	Hazard ratio

HR-CT	High-resolution computer tomography
IBD	Inflammatory bowel disease
IgA	Immunglobulin A
IL	Interleukin
ILD	Interstitial lung disease
INH	Isoniazide
INX	Infliximab
ITT	Intention to treat
IXE	Ixekizumab
JAK	Janus kinase
JIA	Juvenile idiopathic arthritis
LDA	Low disease activity
LDH	Lactate dehydrogenase
LEF	Leflunomide
MCTD	Mixed connective tissue disorder
mg	Milligrams
MISS	Methotrexate intolerance severity score
MPA	Microscopic polyangiitis
MTHFR	Methylene tetrahydrofolate reductase
mTSS	Modified total Sharp score
MTX	Methotrexate
MTX-IR	Insufficient response to MTX
NMSC	Non-melanoma skin cancer
NNT	Number needed to treat
NSAR	Non-steroidal antirheumatic drugs
OA	Oligoarthritis at onset of disease
OR	Odds ratio
PASI	Psoriasis area and severity index
PCFT	Proton-coupled folate transporter
persOA	Persistent oligoarthritis
PG	Polyglutamate
PM	Polymyositis
PsA	Psoriatic arthritis
PUVA	Psoralene plus UV-A
RA	Rheumatoid arthritis
RF	Rheumatoid factor
RFC	Reduced folate carrier
RTX	Rituximab
SAE	Serious adverse events
SAR	Sarilumab
SJC	Swollen joint count
SLE	Systemic lupus erythematodes
SMR	Standardised mortality rate
SSc	Systemic sclerosis
SSZ	Sulfasalazine
TA	Transaminases
TBC	Tuberculosis
TCZ	Tocilizumab
TFB	Tofacitinib
THF	Tetrahydrofolate
TJC	Tender joint count
TNF	Tumor necrosis factor
TOZ	Tocilizumab
TS	Thymidylate synthestase
tsDMARD	Targeted synthetic disease-modifying anti-rheumatic drug
TSS	Total Sharp score
TT	Triple therapy
UE	Unwanted events
UV, UV-A, UV-B	Ultraviolet, ...-A, -B
UPA	Upadacitinib
UST	Ustekinumab
vdH-Score	van der Heijde score
VDZ	Vedolizumab

Table 12.1: Selection of abbreviations used in this book.

Index

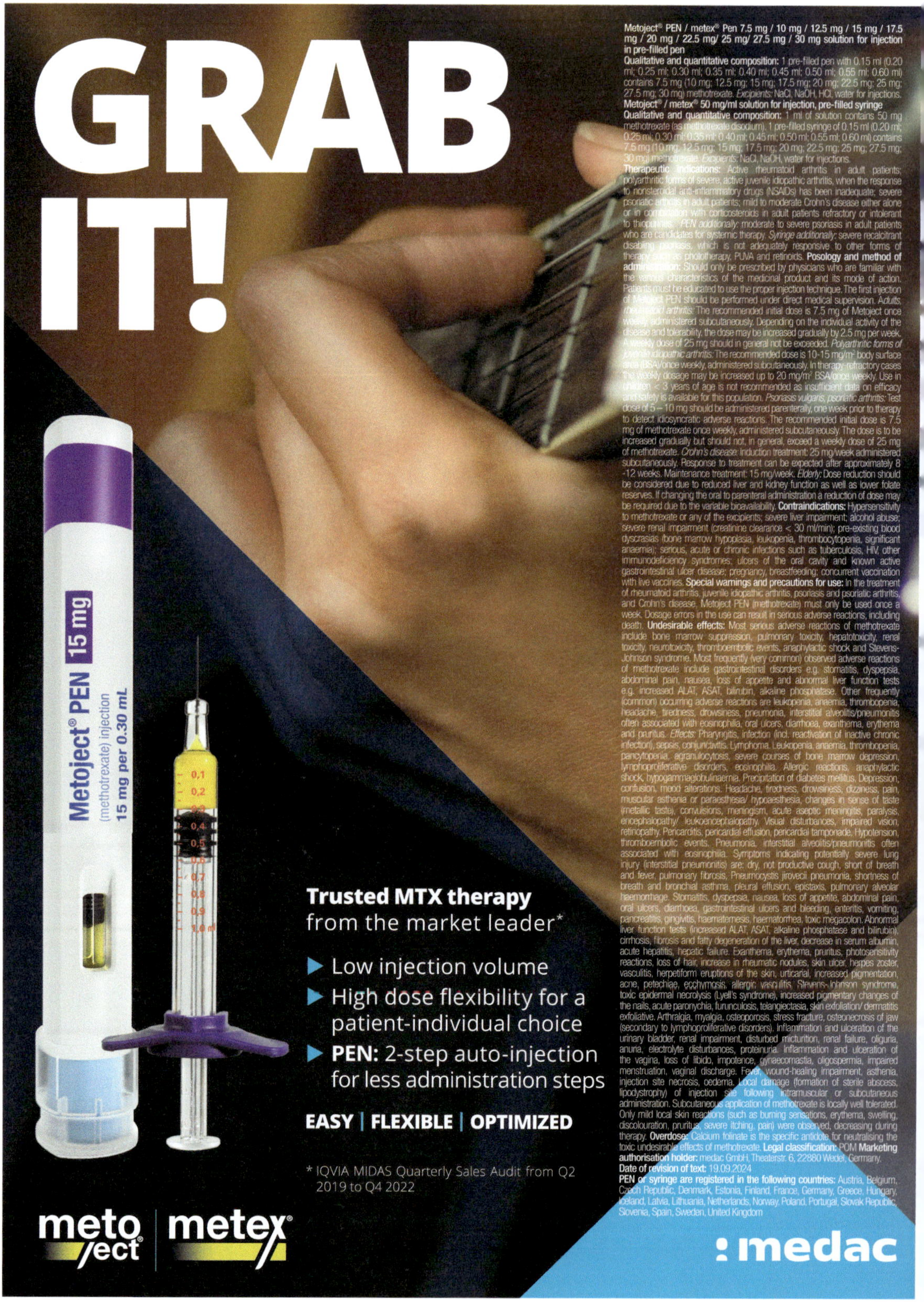
GRAB IT!
Metoject® PEN 15 mg
(methotrexate) injection
15 mg per 0.30 mL
Trusted MTX therapy
from the market leader*
▶ Low injection volume
▶ High dose flexibility for a patient-individual choice
▶ PEN: 2-step auto-injection for less administration steps
EASY | FLEXIBLE | OPTIMIZED
* IQVIA MIDAS Quarterly Sales Audit from Q2 2019 to Q4 2022
meto ject®
metex®
Metoject® PEN / metex® Pen 7.5 mg / 10 mg / 12.5 mg / 15 mg / 17.5 mg / 20 mg / 22.5 mg/ 25 mg/ 27.5 mg / 30 mg solution for injection in pre-filled pen
Qualitative and quantitative composition: 1 pre-filled pen with 0.15 ml (0.20 ml; 0.25 ml; 0.30 ml; 0.35 ml; 0.40 ml; 0.45 ml; 0.50 ml; 0.55 ml; 0.60 ml) contains 7.5 mg (10 mg; 12.5 mg; 15 mg; 17.5 mg; 20 mg; 22.5 mg; 25 mg; 27.5 mg; 30 mg) methotrexate. *Excipients:* NaCl, NaOH, HCl, water for injections.
Metoject® / metex® 50 mg/ml solution for injection, pre-filled syringe
Qualitative and quantitative composition: 1 ml of solution contains 50 mg methotrexate (as methotrexate disodium). 1 pre-filled syringe of 0.15 ml (0.20 ml; 0.25 ml; 0.30 ml; 0.35 ml; 0.40 ml; 0.45 ml; 0.50 ml; 0.55 ml; 0.60 ml) contains 7.5 mg (10 mg; 12.5 mg; 15 mg; 17.5 mg; 20 mg; 22.5 mg; 25 mg; 27.5 mg; 30 mg) methotrexate. *Excipients:* NaCl, NaOH, water for injections.
Therapeutic indications: Active rheumatoid arthritis in adult patients; polyarthritic forms of severe, active juvenile idiopathic arthritis, when the response to nonsteroidal anti-inflammatory drugs (NSAIDs) has been inadequate; severe psoriatic arthritis in adult patients; mild to moderate Crohn's disease either alone or in combination with corticosteroids in adult patients refractory or intolerant to thiopurines. *PEN additionally:* moderate to severe psoriasis in adult patients who are candidates for systemic therapy. *Syringe additionally:* severe recalcitrant disabling psoriasis, which is not adequately responsive to other forms of therapy such as phototherapy, PUVA and retinoids. **Posology and method of administration:** Should only be prescribed by physicians who are familiar with the various characteristics of the medicinal product and its mode of action. Patients must be educated to use the proper injection technique. The first injection of Metoject PEN should be performed under direct medical supervision. *Adults, rheumatoid arthritis:* The recommended initial dose is 7.5 mg of Metoject once weekly, administered subcutaneously. Depending on the individual activity of the disease and tolerability, the dose may be increased gradually by 2.5 mg per week. A weekly dose of 25 mg should in general not be exceeded. *Polyarthritic forms of juvenile idiopathic arthritis:* The recommended dose is 10-15 mg/m² body surface area (BSA)/once weekly, administered subcutaneously. In therapy-refractory cases the weekly dosage may be increased up to 20 mg/m² BSA/once weekly. Use in children < 3 years of age is not recommended as insufficient data on efficacy and safety is available for this population. *Psoriasis vulgaris, psoriatic arthritis:* Test dose of 5 – 10 mg should be administered parenterally, one week prior to therapy to detect idiosyncratic adverse reactions. The recommended initial dose is 7.5 mg of methotrexate once weekly, administered subcutaneously. The dose is to be increased gradually but should not, in general, exceed a weekly dose of 25 mg of methotrexate. *Crohn's disease:* Induction treatment: 25 mg/week administered subcutaneously. Response to treatment can be expected after approximately 8 -12 weeks. Maintenance treatment: 15 mg/week. *Elderly:* Dose reduction should be considered due to reduced liver and kidney function as well as lower folate reserves. If changing the oral to parenteral administration a reduction of dose may be required due to the variable bioavailability. **Contraindications:** Hypersensitivity to methotrexate or any of the excipients; severe liver impairment; alcohol abuse; severe renal impairment (creatinine clearance < 30 ml/min); pre-existing blood dyscrasias (bone marrow hypoplasia, leukopenia, thrombocytopenia, significant anaemia); serious, acute or chronic infections such as tuberculosis, HIV, other immunodeficiency syndromes; ulcers of the oral cavity and known active gastrointestinal ulcer disease; pregnancy, breastfeeding; concurrent vaccination with live vaccines. **Special warnings and precautions for use:** In the treatment of rheumatoid arthritis, juvenile idiopathic arthritis, psoriasis and psoriatic arthritis, and Crohn's disease, Metoject PEN (methotrexate) must only be used once a week. Dosage errors in the use can result in serious adverse reactions, including death. **Undesirable effects:** Most serious adverse reactions of methotrexate include bone marrow suppression, pulmonary toxicity, hepatotoxicity, renal toxicity, neurotoxicity, thromboembolic events, anaphylactic shock and Stevens-Johnson syndrome. Most frequently (very common) observed adverse reactions of methotrexate include gastrointestinal disorders e.g. stomatitis, dyspepsia, abdominal pain, nausea, loss of appetite and abnormal liver function tests e.g. increased ALAT, ASAT, bilirubin, alkaline phosphatase. Other frequently (common) occurring adverse reactions are leukopenia, anaemia, thrombopenia, headache, tiredness, drowsiness, pneumonia, interstitial alveolitis/pneumonitis often associated with eosinophilia, oral ulcers, diarrhoea, exanthema, erythema and pruritus. *Effects:* Pharyngitis, infection (incl. reactivation of inactive chronic infection), sepsis, conjunctivitis. Lymphoma. Leukopenia, anaemia, thrombopenia, pancytopenia, agranulocytosis, severe courses of bone marrow depression, lymphoproliferative disorders, eosinophilia. Allergic reactions, anaphylactic shock, hypogammaglobulinaemia. Precipitation of diabetes mellitus. Depression, confusion, mood alterations. Headache, tiredness, drowsiness, dizziness, pain, muscular asthenia or paraesthesia/ hypoaesthesia, changes in sense of taste (metallic taste), convulsions, meningism, acute aseptic meningitis, paralysis, encephalopathy/ leukoencephalopathy. Visual disturbances, impaired vision, retinopathy. Pericarditis, pericardial effusion, pericardial tamponade. Hypotension, thromboembolic events. Pneumonia, interstitial alveolitis/pneumonitis often associated with eosinophilia. Symptoms indicating potentially severe lung injury (interstitial pneumonitis) are: dry, not productive cough, short of breath and fever, pulmonary fibrosis, Pneumocystis jirovecii pneumonia, shortness of breath and bronchial asthma, pleural effusion, epistaxis, pulmonary alveolar haemorrhage. Stomatitis, dyspepsia, nausea, loss of appetite, abdominal pain, oral ulcers, diarrhoea, gastrointestinal ulcers and bleeding, enteritis, vomiting, pancreatitis, gingivitis, haematemesis, haematorrhea, toxic megacolon. Abnormal liver function tests (increased ALAT, ASAT, alkaline phosphatase and bilirubin), cirrhosis, fibrosis and fatty degeneration of the liver, decrease in serum albumin, acute hepatitis, hepatic failure. Exanthema, erythema, pruritus, photosensitivity reactions, loss of hair, increase in rheumatic nodules, skin ulcer, herpes zoster, vasculitis, herpetiform eruptions of the skin, urticarial, increased pigmentation, acne, petechiae, ecchymosis, allergic vasculitis, Stevens-Johnson syndrome, toxic epidermal necrolysis (Lyell's syndrome), increased pigmentary changes of the nails, acute paronychia, furunculosis, telangiectasia, skin exfoliation/ dermatitis exfoliative. Arthralgia, myalgia, osteoporosis, stress fracture, osteonecrosis of jaw (secondary to lymphoproliferative disorders). Inflammation and ulceration of the urinary bladder, renal impairment, disturbed micturition, renal failure, oliguria, anuria, electrolyte disturbances, proteinuria. Inflammation and ulceration of the vagina, loss of libido, impotence, gynaecomastia, oligospermia, impaired menstruation, vaginal discharge. Fever, wound-healing impairment, asthenia, injection site necrosis, oedema. Local damage (formation of sterile abscess, lipodystrophy) of injection site following intramuscular or subcutaneous administration. Subcutaneous application of methotrexate is locally well tolerated. Only mild local skin reactions (such as burning sensations, erythema, swelling, discolouration, pruritus, severe itching, pain) were observed, decreasing during therapy. **Overdose:** Calcium folinate is the specific antidote for neutralising the toxic undesirable effects of methotrexate. **Legal classification:** POM **Marketing authorisation holder:** medac GmbH, Theaterstr. 6, 22880 Wedel, Germany.
Date of revision of text: 19.09.2024
PEN or syringe are registered in the following countries: Austria, Belgium, Czech Republic, Denmark, Estonia, Finland, France, Germany, Greece, Hungary, Iceland, Latvia, Lithuania, Netherlands, Norway, Poland, Portugal, Slovak Republic, Slovenia, Spain, Sweden, United Kingdom
: medac